Exercise Prescription for Medical Conditions

Medical Conditions

Handbook for Physical Therapists

Exercise Prescription
for Medical Conditions

Handbook for
Physical Therapists

Catherine Goodman, PT, MBA, CBP
Medical Multimedia Group, Medical Writer
University of Montana
School of Pharmacy and Allied Health Sciences
Department of Physical Therapy
Faculty Affiliate
Missoula, MT

Kevin Helgeson, PT, DHSc
Rocky Mountain University of Health Professions
Provo, UT

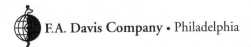 F.A. Davis Company • Philadelphia

F. A. Davis Company
1915 Arch Street
Philadelphia, PA 19103
www.fadavis.com

Printed in the United States of America

Last digit indicates print number: 10 9 8 7 6 5 4 3 2 1

Publisher: Margaret M. Biblis
Manager of Content Development: George W. Lang
Developmental Editor: Peg Waltner
Manager of Art and Design: Carolyn O'Brien

As new scientific information becomes available through basic and clinical research, recommended treatments and drug therapies undergo changes. The author(s) and publisher have done everything possible to make this book accurate, up to date, and in accord with accepted standards at the time of publication. The author(s), editors, and publisher are not responsible for errors or omissions or for consequences from application of the book, and make no warranty, expressed or implied, in regard to the contents of the book. Any practice described in this book should be applied by the reader in accordance with professional standards of care used in regard to the unique circumstances that may apply in each situation. The reader is advised always to check product information (package inserts) for changes and new information regarding dose and contraindications before administering any drug. Caution is especially urged when using new or infrequently ordered drugs.

*To Ed and Sandy, for their loving
example
To Loriann, for standing beside
me for the long run
and to Connor and Colin, for the joy
they bring us both*
KMH

PREFACE

Every educator (the authors included) is cautious about prescribing any intervention in a cookbook fashion. But there comes a time in a clinician's life when researching evidence-based exercise protocols for each client or even groups of clients becomes impossible. This is especially true when new information and ideas on the topic are being published with increasing frequency.

Additionally, everyone needs a starting point. The goal of this book is to provide you, the physical therapist, with that starting point for exercise for clients, based on their primary medical (not physical therapy) diagnosis and various comorbidities present. This text offers a review and compilation of the literature to date and provides a consensus on approaches to exercise for each disease entity discussed.

Physicians may use what looks like a "cookbook-like" approach with medical or surgical procedures. Physicians call these "protocols" and, as often as possible, these treatment protocols are developed as a result of research compiling evidence focused on outcomes. Establishing accepted protocols is an important way to provide evidence-based practice and develop guidelines that can be modified as further evidence regarding outcomes is published.

Educators want students to understand the reasoning behind (for example) the causes and management of anemia so that students can create their own exercise prescriptions. This is certainly not an evidence-based approach, although it is a reasonable way to practice when the literature does not offer any alternative information.

Exercise is being recognized more and more as an important modality to use in gaining good health and in recovering from illness and disease. Research supports the notion that exercise is an effective intervention for many diseases, illnesses, and conditions. But what kind of exercise is best? How much? How often? At what intensity? The physical therapist is uniquely qualified to prescribe exercise as an intervention for medical disease, given the understanding of pathology, physiology, biomechanics, and exercise. In order to prescribe the most appropriate and most effective exercise for each condition, evidence-based knowledge of these parameters is important.

This text is an attempt to give you, the physical therapist, the most up-to-date information from which to start in prescribing exercise specifically to treat medical conditions. General concepts of disease and exercise should be used to modify these "prescriptions." The exercise types—their intensity, duration, and frequency—presented here are merely guidelines to get you started. Granted, the volume, breadth, and depth of evidence is fairly lacking at this time. You will see that reflected in the lack of specific parameters for many conditions reported in this text. We feel certain that, in time, the research will expand, broaden, and reflect the change in focus from treatment to prevention of medical conditions. We intend to keep abreast of those changes and keep you apprised of those changes with subsequent editions of this text.

Some may wonder how this text is different from the American College of Sports Medicine's (ACSM) *Exercise Management for Persons with Chronic Diseases and Disabilities.* There are two main differences. First, this text is more of a quick reference, reflective of results of studies reported in the current literature. Second, we deal more with systemic diseases, whereas the ACSM's text covers more of the traditional orthopedic, neurologic, cardiopulmonary, and neuromuscular disorders.

Physical therapists are practicing under direct access in a majority of the states, with the eventual goal of all 50 states becoming direct access states. This policy has influenced the profession in its move to develop entry-level doctorate programs. A doctor of physical therapy (DPT) is, indeed, the best health-care professional to assess human movement impairments and the physical needs of each client/patient to develop a plan of care, including an exercise prescription.

Along with a DPT level of education, the American Physical Therapy Association (APTA) is positioning physical therapists to become primary care therapists. This means we are the first (and sometimes only) health-care professional to evaluate and treat the client. In this expanded role, advanced competencies such as described in this text will be quite appropriate.

The APTA has also directed physical therapists to include primary, secondary, and tertiary prevention as part of our intervention whenever appropriate and possible. As more and more research shows the importance of exercise in fostering wellness and in preventing and treating various diseases, conditions, and illnesses, the focus will shift from a rehabilitation approach to a wellness/prevention approach. The need for information of this kind is already present and will only increase in the coming years.

This text does *not* provide exercise prescriptions or protocols for neuromuscular or musculoskeletal conditions. It is designed to discuss exercise in the prevention and treatment of medical diseases, conditions, and illnesses such as cancer, heart disease, thyroid conditions, liver impairment, anemia, lupus, and so on.

At the present time our profession focuses on treating neurologic and orthopedic clients who also have comorbidities. The future of physical therapy will need to include clients seeking physical therapy as the primary intervention for all medical conditions when appropriate.

Regarding the need to include a pediatric focus, it seems that children always get left out. Most research in this topic area at this time is geared toward adults. Many diseases present in adults are not present in the pediatric population. The possible exceptions are cystic fibrosis and cancer. Research in pediatric groups is problematic for ethical reasons. Children tend to recover faster and with less intervention; activity is emphasized, but specific exercise protocols are not the focus of research efforts. We included information that was relevant in populations groups under age 18 whenever it was available.

Progression of exercise programs will be necessary, but right now the research is based on foundational programs and has not begun to investigate the effects of progression or even how to progress. We hope topics like prescriptive exercise for medical disease and progression of exercise will become the focus of research by physical therapists in the very near future.

Catherine C. Goodman
Kevin M. Helgeson

Michael Chiacchiero, PT, DPT
Assistant Professor
College of Staten Island
Staten Island, NY

Susan A. Chinworth, PhD, PT
Associate Professor
Physical Therapy Education
Elon University
Elon, NC

Deanna Dye, PT, PhD
Assistant Professor
Idaho State University
Pocatello, ID

Dawn T. Gulick, PhD, PT, ATC, CSCS
Associate Professor
Physical Therapy
Widener University
Chester, PA

Reed Humphrey, PhD, PT
Professor and Chair
School of Physical Therapy and
Rehabilitation Science
University of Montana
Missoula, MT

Scott Marek, DPT
Outpatient Clinical Coordinator
St. Luke's Sports and Rehabilitation
Blakeslee, PA

Jaime C. Paz, PT, MS
Associate Clinical Specialist
Physical Therapy
Northeastern University
Boston, MA

Jeffrey Rothman, PT, EdD
Director
Physical Therapy
City University of New York
Staten Island, NY

Elizabeth L. Weiss, PhD, PT
Department Head, Professor
Physical Therapy
Louisiana State University
New Orleans, LA

Philip L. Witt, PhD, PT
Associate Professor
Allied Health Science
University of North Carolina,
Chapel Hill, NC

CONTENTS

Introduction

Introduction to Physical Activity and Exercise for the Medically Compromised Patient

Benefits of Physical Activity and Exercise

Exercise is the most powerful "wonder" drug in the United States. In fact, the American College of Sports Medicine (ACSM) has launched a program called "Exercise is Medicine," with the sole purpose of getting Americans to incorporate physical activity and exercise into their daily routine, especially those with health problems.[1]

ACSM has called on physicians to prescribe exercise to their clients and then assess and review every client's physical activity program at every visit. "Exercise is Medicine" aims to make physical activity and exercise a standard part of disease prevention and treatment in the United States. Physicians are encouraged to record physical activity and exercise as a vital sign. One of the goals of the program is to increase collaborations among physicians and exercise professionals, including physical therapists, to benefit people for whom exercise and increased physical activity can prevent, treat, or manage chronic diseases.

Exercise has proved effective in the primary and secondary prevention and treatment of more than 25 diseases and chronic conditions. Decades of science confirm that exercise improves health and can extend life expectancy. Type 2 diabetes, breast and colon cancer, hypertension, heart disease, obesity, depression, osteoporosis, chronic obstructive pulmonary disease, and arthritis comprise a partial list of the conditions and illnesses that can be affected by exercise. Regular activity can improve the quality of life and general well-being and mood, reduce stress, improve sleep, sharpen cognitive function, and improve sexual function.

Studies consistently show a benefit in general health and aerobic fitness via exercise training. Randomized controlled trials examining the effects of different intensities and amounts of exercise on peak oxygen consumption (Vo_2 max) make it clear that fitness levels are improved even with low amounts of exercise. Although the effect of exercise alone is substantial, it is significantly magnified when accompanied by other lifestyle changes, such as good nutrition and weight loss. Just burning calories through exercise is a beneficial side effect.[2]

It is appropriate to recommend mild exercise to improve fitness and reduce cardiovascular risk while also encouraging higher intensities and amounts for additional benefit.[3,4] Even a single weekly bout of high-intensity exercise has been shown effective in reducing the risk of death in groups of adults with known cardiovascular disease compared with those who reported no activity.[5]

Light to moderate exercise has been shown to limit the damaging effects of excess free radical formation now linked to a wide range of diseases. Regular physical activity and exercise have been linked to a reduction in mortality from all causes; just one exercise session weekly can make a difference.[6,7] Even knowing this, the majority of adults in the United States are not physically active at levels that can promote health.[8]

The acute effects of exercise have been proved: levels of serum triglycerides are reduced for up to 72 hours after exercise, systolic blood pressure is reduced for up to 12 hours, improvements in insulin sensitivity are made, glucose homeostasis is normalized, C-reactive protein linked with the risk of cardiovascular complications is reduced,[9] and high-density lipoprotein cholesterol can be raised. But these effects are transient (temporary); thus, the recommendation for adults to participate in moderate-intensity physical activity 5 to 7 days a week.[10,11]

The effects of acute exercise on platelet reactivity are also well known. Long-term endurance physical training at moderate intensity (50%–74% of maximal oxygen consumption or Vo_2 max) suppresses platelet adhesiveness and aggregation (thus lowering the risk of vascular thrombosis) both at rest and after acute strenuous exercise. The effects reverse back to the pretraining state after a period of deconditioning, emphasizing the importance of regular moderate exercise.[12,13]

Putting Wellness and Fitness First: The Prevention Approach to Health

How ironic that this message arrives at a time when the United States has become the most sedentary nation in the world. Obesity is at epidemic levels, while armchair wellness is sweeping the nation.

People may know nutrition, physical activity, and exercise are the keys to better health, but their taste buds have been tuned to salty and sweet, and their preferences are for high-fat foods. There is also a microwave mentality: picture yourself standing in front of the microwave, arms folded across your chest, toe tapping impatiently as you say to yourself, "Come on, come on, come on. I don't have all minute."

It is fitting that U.S. society with urgency as its emblem should have such a dependence on its addictions and drugs to get through the day, whether those are alcohol, work, chocolate or other "comfort" foods, and drugs from Prozac to Valium.

Often, someone is overweight and depressed. At age 50, blood pressure is starting to creep up. Maybe the individual has been diagnosed with fibromyalgia but has had asthma since childhood. Maybe he or she is recovering from cancer or has a significant family history of cancer and wants to do something to prevent it occurring personally. Just what kind of exercise should the person do? What kind of advice do you give your clients with similar stories?

The scientific community is actively researching exercise and its impact on individual diseases. Findings such as the fact that exercise capacity is an independent predictor of mortality in women catch the attention of the news media, which then alert the general population.[14] Exercise before surgery has a proven benefit in reducing hospital stay and eliminating a prolonged recovery time.[15] For many individuals, exercise is significantly more effective than medication for type 2 diabetes, even making it possible to maintain proper glucose levels without medications; for others, regular exercise helps manage the condition more effectively along with medications.[16] This is a sample of the type of evidence already available that will eventually convince insurers to cover "prehabilitation" programs.

Research on the topic of prescriptive exercise is ongoing. How do our clients apply this information to their daily lives? Where do they get the kind of information they need for their particular health background and current concerns? Who can dispense exercise prescription? Physical therapists, of course!

As the American Physical Therapy Association positions physical therapists as *the* experts in restoring and improving motion in people's lives, we are promoting physical activity that goes beyond function and bringing a fitness and wellness perspective to the services we offer.[17]

Health-Care Reform

Health-care reform has been the topic of many news reports, legislative and presidential debates, and health-care organizations for the last decade. There has been an increasing emphasis on a health-care system focused on prevention and wellness rather than on illness and treatment. The health-care community, third-party payers, and even the government are already beginning to reframe health as wellness first, rather than medical care. A paradigm shift is in process from a disease-based model to a prevention-based approach that is proactive, rather than reactive.

Legislative measures to strengthen the role of primary care and chronic care management have been introduced.[18] During Senate confirmation hearings for the secretary of the U.S. Department of Health and Human Services, nominees discussed issues that could have an effect on health-care reform and physical therapy, including prevention and wellness. APTA continues to follow and report on health-care reform as it relates to prevention and wellness. Updates can be accessed at the APTA Health Care Reform Center (www.apta.org; type "health care reform center" in the Search box).

In the near future, the goal will be to assess individuals for optimal lifestyle strategies and provide the necessary support to achieve them. Encouraging physical activity and exercise is a very effective way to reduce health-care costs in all age groups, but especially older Americans. Even Medicare has expressed an interest in developing a plan to cover the costs of lifestyle modifications, such as exercise, that have a proven benefit to their recipients.[19]

This text will help therapists positioned to step into this role quickly and easily, as the health-care delivery system will increasingly demand these kinds of services.

The Role of the Physical Therapist

APTA has a new position on promoting physical activity/exercise, which amends HOD P06-03-29-28 and underlines the benefits of physical activity/exercise and the role of the physical therapist in promoting those benefits. The position calls for APTA to endorse appropriate physical activity/exercise goals and objectives put forth by government and other nationally recognized agencies; support and encourage APTA members to provide leadership in supporting scientific, educational, and legislative activities directed to the promotion of regular physical activity/exercise in order to enhance health and prevent disease; and encourage members to adopt healthy lifestyle choices that include meeting national guidelines for participating in physical activity/exercise.[20]

APTA supports providing services for two groups of individuals: those with health issues and those at risk for health issues. The physical therapist can create a plan specific to them, while continuing to promote a role in health, wellness, and fitness for all populations.

The plan includes definitions and clarifications of terms associated with health, wellness, and fitness. For example, Goal II states: "Physical therapists are universally recognized and promoted as providers of fitness, health promotion, wellness, and risk reduction programs to enhance quality of life for persons across the life-span."[21] Four main objectives associated with this plan include:

Objective A: Enhance the ability of physical therapists to provide services that positively affect fitness, promote health and wellness, and foster risk reduction across the life span.
Objective B: Enhance the quality of physical therapy education in fitness, health promotion, wellness, and risk reduction across the life span.
Objective C: Disseminate evidence to internal and external stakeholders about practice in fitness, health promotion, wellness, and risk reduction across the life span.
Objective D: Promote physical therapists as practitioners of choice for fitness, health promotion, wellness, and risk reduction across the life span.

Physical therapists are uniquely positioned to combine their understanding of the pathology of underlying diseases and illnesses along with their knowledge of physiology and its relation to exercise. In the context of preventing or treating chronic illnesses, diseases, and other systemic conditions, the terms "prescriptive exercise" or "exercise prescription" are fairly new. Clinicians faced with individuals who have orthopedic and neurologic along with multiple comorbidities are looking for this information. Clients of all ages, but especially those in the Baby Boom generation (born between 1946 and 1964), are asking, "I have X, Y or Z disease. Or I have a family history of X, Y, or Z condition. What's the best exercise program for me?"

Therapists are studying isolated diseases, trying to answer this question one case at a time. For example, every day physical therapists in acute care, home health, and outpatient rehabilitation are faced with the question: "What's the best exercise for someone with a total hip who also has hypertension (or diabetes, or thyroiditis, or pancreatitis, or any other comorbidity present)?" There is no definitive text to guide the therapist when making decisions about the right exercise for someone who has other health conditions outside the neuromuscular or musculoskeletal system. So let's get started meeting the need!

Considerations, Precautions, and Contraindications

Considerations

As with strength training programs, any exercise program must take into consideration the client's current health, past medical history, lifestyle, risk factors, and orthopedic and neurologic condition. Limitations that may be aggravated by exercise training (frequency, intensity, duration) must be factored into the exercise prescription. Anemia, low testosterone levels, low hematocrit/hemoglobin levels, and sarcopenia (loss of muscle strength and mass) are just a few of the biologic factors that can affect the ability to complete any form of exercise.

Motivation and Compliance

Despite the fact that the focus of clinical care is changing from cure to prevention, motivating people to increase their activity level can be a challenge. Compliance with conventional exercise regimens is often low. For those who respond to a prescribed program, initial enthusiasm is often followed by a lapse or discontinuation of the activity. Benefits are not always realized; for example, some people will never know the disease or condition was prevented by exercise. So, there is a certain amount of faith in the process based on statistical models that may be more motivating for some than for others.

The individual's current health should always be taken into consideration. In older adults, this may be due to health factors that limit exercise, lack of motivation, and inability to sustain long-term interest among other reasons.[22,23]

Researchers looking for factors that influence exercise behavior have investigated multiple factors as contributors or constraints, including environmental influences, genetic contributions, socioeconomic status, access to exercise facilities, job issues, time constraints, injuries, and health beliefs. Injuries, especially, create a barrier to participation in older age groups. Poor compliance is also more likely when the client has had some types of strokes or is using muscle relaxants, sedatives, or other medications that can reduce desire or drive to exercise.

For individuals with chronic pain or problems like fibromyalgia or chronic fatigue syndrome, symptoms of pain and fatigue increase during exercise, resulting in limited compliance and limited long-term benefits. The therapist can explain that pain may result in part from muscle spasm and reduced blood flow to muscles, both of which can be aided by persistence in managing exercise.

Using training intensity as a measure of improvement may be helpful. Before performing the physical activity or exercise, compute the maximum heart rate (MHR = 220 – age). During the activity/exercise, take the pulse, and record this for later calculations.

Once the activity/exercise is completed, compute the intensity of work: I_W = Pulse/MHR. Multiply I_W by the number of minutes exercised to determine the Training Index (TI) [TI = I_W × number of minutes]. Keep track of the TI for each activity/exercise session, and total them for 1 week. Track this value over time to assess improved outcomes.

Understanding how to motivate people to seek lifelong healthy behaviors (including exercise) requires a working familiarity with the social, behavioral, and psychologic components of decision making in the context of changing behavior. For example, therapists can help clients identify and target unhealthy or unhelpful behaviors and replace them with behaviors that promote health and prevent illness. Encouraging self-efficacy as a way to help people gain self-confidence in their ability to control their symptoms and to understand how their health problems affect their lives is important. Resources are available to help (e.g., Stanford Patient Education Research Center, Stanford University, http://patienteducation.stanford.edu/).

The plan of care must include interventions that are safe, enjoyable, accessible, and match the client's stage of change. One model that addresses this approach is the Stages of Change or Transtheoretical Model.[24] This model proposes these stages: precontemplation, contemplation, preparation, action, and maintenance. In the *precontemplation* stage, the person has no intention of changing and/or is unaware of the problem or risk associated with the behavior. In the *contemplation* stage, the individual is aware of the problem and may consider change but has no specific plans (or commitment) to do so. In this stage, the person may feel or say he or she is "stuck." *Preparation* requires an attitude that says, "I am planning to take action soon." In fact, the person may have tried to do so already but failed to achieve the desired goal. *Action* is characterized by taking specific steps to address the behavior change desired. Change is not yet consistent at this point. The therapist has a key role in helping individuals reach the action stage as quickly as possible and committing to *maintain* (maintenance) or stay in that stage for a lifetime.

Another consideration must include the needs of chronically disabled children and adults who are mobility-challenged and have a limited capacity for physical activity. Therapists can be very instrumental in identifying the unique needs of this population and finding ways to help them improve their fitness level.

Genetics

There appears to be a substantial genetic contribution to exercise behavior. Some people seem to find the acute effects of exercise more pleasurable than others. This suggests there may be possible ways to create more successful interventions and motivate participation in exercise programs.[25]

Precautions

Although the dangers of inactivity are the primary focus of this text, there are some dangers in being active, especially for those participating in sports and repetitive activities.

Sports injuries affect individuals of all ages. Physical therapists play an important role in recognizing potential harm and preventing injuries or reinjuries.

One area of potential concern is the repetitive and prolonged pressures applied to the plantar aspect of the feet during running (especially in stair climbing, elliptical training, or other similar activity). High-impact forces can lead to orthopedic conditions such as metatarsal stress fractures or foot ulcers in anyone with sensory neuropathies (e.g., diabetes, post chemotherapy). Susceptible individuals must be evaluated and monitored with careful and appropriate selection of exercises. Age-related variations in ground-reaction force patterns and foot structure can also increase the risk of damage from high pressures.[26]

Interval training with alternate bursts of intense activity and periods of rest or gentler activity works for a wide range of cardiovascular conditions, such as stable coronary artery disease, intermittent claudication, heart failure, and diabetes. Early work on interval training for chronic conditions conducted by cardiologist Dr. Vojin Smodlaka[27,28] has been followed up by a few recent studies. In all studies so far (animals and humans), interval training had better outcomes when compared with continuous exercise for these conditions.[29,30]

Data from the Physicians' Health study suggests that vigorous exercise (defined as 30 minutes of six metabolic equivalents [METs] or more) could increase the risk of sudden death in sedentary individuals who are not accustomed to regular physical stress.[31] Whereas regular exercise and activity is protective in lowering the risk of coronary heart disease, sudden, vigorous exercise can result in sudden death during and up to 30 minutes after vigorous exertion. Anyone with pre-existing atherosclerotic vascular (or other heart) disease and other sedentary individuals who are susceptible are at risk. The proposed mechanisms for this response are available but remain outside the scope of this text.[32]

The therapist prescribing and supervising an exercise program for individuals with poor fitness, deconditioned status, the presence of heart or lung disease, or other comorbidities must be aware of the person's physiologic limits to exercise. For example, people with congestive heart failure have reduced blood flow to muscles, which contributes to their reduced exercise capacity. However, their central dysfunction is not a contraindication to peripheral exercise. Even a mild change in peripheral perfusion can dramatically change morbidity and mortality risk.[33,34]

Medications can affect cardiac output and limit maximal heart rate. Hyperventilation can occur in individuals with conditions associated with muscle weakness or disorders of muscle metabolism. In people with cardiac disorders, perceived effort with exercise (based on breathing) is greater than someone of the same age and body type who does not have cardiac compromise. Shortness of breath in anyone with cardiac or respiratory disease can be very limiting when trying to develop an exercise program.[35] It can take time to slowly increase exercise by increments tolerated by the affected individual. The therapist must remain diligent in documenting changes, encouraging the client, and providing encouragement along the way.

A careful and thorough assessment of the individual is essential. For example, people with pulmonary disorders often quit exercising because it is perceived as "too much work" or "too difficult." The perception of muscle effort and fatigue may not just be the result of poor exercise capacity, poor ventilation, or reduced cardiac output. It could be that skeletal muscle weakness is the primary limitation. The individual may need treatment to improve airflow resistance and/or decreased cardiac output along with a concomitant strength-training program. Addressing all factors that contribute to limited breathing and skeletal muscle activity will increase the chances for keeping the individual exercising and, ultimately, having a successful outcome.[35]

More and more older adults are initiating a program of weight training for themselves without any prior knowledge of lifting or training techniques. Unfortunately, there is a proportional increase in injuries related to weight training. Women are more likely to get safety instruction but less likely to use a spotter or a weight belt compared with men.[36,37] The therapist can be instrumental in initiating or reminding adults engaged in weight training about the use of precautions such as wearing firm traction shoes, stretching properly, and warming up before lifting weights. The therapist can also provide review and supervision of the person's current weight-lifting program.

Contraindications

The therapist must always rely on clinical assessment and personal judgment based on the individual's current health, vital signs, and comorbidities when determining what is or is not a contraindication for exercise therapy. ACSM does a good job of outlining the basic indications and contraindications for exercise prescription; physical therapists have come to rely on this source.[38] A quick summary of contraindications is available (Box 1-1).

Box 1-1 | **Medical Precautions/Contraindications for Exercise Therapy**

- Medically unstable
- Unstable vital signs (acute systemic illness or high fever; severe hypertension [systolic blood pressure greater than 200 mm Hg or resting diastolic greater than 110 mm Hg]; uncontrolled tachycardia [more than 120 bpm])
- Unstable angina
- Unstable aortic aneurysm
- Uncontrolled arrhythmias
- Uncompensated congestive heart failure
- Uncontrolled or unstable blood glucose <80–100 mg/dL or >250–400 mg/dL; these values can vary from individual to individual)*
- Severe dehydration or heat stroke (e.g., watch for postural hypotension, dizziness, confusion, poor skin turgor, low urine output)
- Severe anemia
- Low oxygen saturation (<95% requires evaluation; <90% for anyone with COPD)

Data from American College of Sports Medicine: Resource Manual for Guidelines for Exercise Testing and Prescription, 6/e. Philadelphia, 2009.

*Exercise may need to be postponed until safe blood glucose levels are achieved.

Summary

Exercise as a successful intervention for many diseases, illness, and conditions will become prescriptive as research shows how much and what kind of exercise can prevent or mediate each problem. There is already a great deal of information on this topic as well as an accompanying need to change the way people think about exercise.

Convincing people to establish lifelong patterns of exercise and physical activity will continue to be a major focus of the health-care industry. Therapists can advocate disease prevention, wellness, and promotion of healthy lifestyles by delivering health-care services intended to prevent health problems or maintain health and by offering annual wellness screening and exercise prescription aimed at reducing or eliminating risk factors as part of primary care prevention.

References

1. Sallis RE: Exercise is medicine program. American College of Sports Medicine. Available at www.acsm.org. See also www.exerciseismedicine.org. Accessed January 14, 2009.
2. Fletcher G, Trejo JF: Why and how to prescribe exercise: Overcoming the barriers. Cleveland Clin J Med 72(8):645-656, 2005.
3. Johnson JL: Exercise training amount and intensity effects on metabolic syndrome: Studies of a targeted risk reduction intervention through defined exercise (STRRIDE). Am J Cardiol 100(12):1759-1766, 2007.
4. Slentz CA: Inactivity, exercise training and detraining, and plasma lipoproteins: STRRIDE: A randomized, controlled study of exercise intensity and amount. J Appl Physiol 103(2):432-442, 2007.
5. Wisloff U: A single weekly bout of exercise may reduce cardiovascular mortality: How little pain for cardiac gain? The HUNT study, Norway. Eur J Cardiovasc Prev Rehabil 13(5):798-804, 2006.
6. Moholdt T: Physical activity and mortality in men and women with coronary heart disease: A prospective population-based cohort study in Norway (the HUNT study). Eur J Cardiovasc Prev Rehabil 15(6): 639-645, 2008.
7. Warburton DE. Health benefits of physical activity: The evidence. CMAJ 174:801-809, 2006.
8. Macera CA: Prevalence of physical activity, including lifestyle activities among adults—United States, 2000-2001. MMWR 53(32):764-769, 2003.
9. Milani RV: Reduction in C-reactive protein through cardiac rehabilitation and exercise training. J Am Coll Cardiol 43:1056-1061, 2004.
10. Pate RR, Pratt M, Blair SN: Physical activity and public health. A recommendation from the Centers for Disease Control and Prevention and the American College of Sports Medicine. JAMA 273:402-407, 1995.
11. Martin SL, Vehige T: Establishing public health benchmarks for physical activity programs [letter to editor]. Prev Chronic Dis [serial online] 2006 Jul [date cited]. Available from http://www.cdc.gov/pcd/issues/2006/jul/06_0006.htm. Accessed December 15, 2008.
12. Lee KW, Lip GYH: Acute versus habitual exercise, thrombogenesis and exercise intensity. Thromb Haemost 91:416-419, 2004.
13. Wang JS: Exercise prescription and thrombogenesis. J Biomed Sci 13(6):753-761, 2006.
14. Gulati M. The prognostic value of a nomogram for exercise capacity in women. NEJM 353(5):468-475, 2005.
15. Brown M, Taylor J: Prehabilitation and rehabilitation for attenuating hindlimb unweighting effects on skeletal muscle and gait in adult and old rats. Arch Phys Med Rehabil 86:2261-2269, 2005.
16. Knowler WC: Reduction of the incidence of type 2 diabetes with lifestyle intervention or metformin. NEJM 346(6):393-403, 2002.
17. Ries E: Well beyond function. PT Magazine 17(5):21-27, 2009.
18. Baucus M: A call to action on healthcare (white paper). Senate Finance Committee Chairman. November 12, 2008. Available at http://finance.senate.gov/healthreform2009/finalwhitepaper.pdf. Accessed January 2, 2009.
19. Jones W: Fifty years from now: Today's baby reaches middle age. In Wallace M: The Way We Will Be 50 Years From Today. Thomas Nelson, Nashville, TN, 2008, pp. 26-30.

20. Physical therapists and physical therapist assistants as promoters and advocates for physical activity/exercise. HOD P06-08-07-08 (Program 32) [Initial HOD P06-03-29-28; RC 2-08] [Previously titled: Promoting Physical Activity] [Position] 12/09/08 Available at http://www.apta.org/AM/Template.cfm?Section= Archives2&Template=/Customsource/TaggedPage/PTIssue.cfm&Issue=06/17/2008#article49315. Accessed August 08, 2009.

21. American Physical Therapy Association: Plan to describe, communicate, and reinforce the physical therapist's role in providing services that improve physical fitness in two priority populations. PT Bulletin Online 6(48), November 15, 2005. Available at www.apta.org/AM/Template.cfm?Section=Archive. Accessed December 15, 2008.

22. Mayoux-Benhamou M: Predictors of compliance with a home-based exercise program added to usual medical care in preventing postmenopausal osteoporosis: An 18-month prospective study. Osteoporosis Int 2005;16:325-331.

23. Wallace B, Cummings R: Systematic review of randomized trials of the effect of exercise on bone mass in pre- and postmenopausal women. Calcif Tissue Int 67:10-18, 2000.

24. Prochaska JO: Changing for Good: A Revolutionary Six-Stage Program for Overcoming Bad Habits and Moving Your Life Positively Forward. Avon Books, New York, 1995.

25. Stubbe JH: Genetic influences on exercise participation in 37,051 twin pairs from seven countries. Plos ONE 1(1):e22, 2006.

26. Burnfield JM: Variations in plantar pressure variables across five cardiovascular exercises. Med Sci Sports Exerc 39(11):2012-2020, 2007.

27. Smodlaka VN: Interval training in rehabilitation medicine. Arch Phys Med Rehabil 54(9):428-431, 1973.

28. Smodlaka VN: Reconditioning of emphysema patients using interval training. N Y State J Med 74(6): 951-955, 1974.

29. Wisloff U: Superior cardiovascular effect of aerobic interval training versus moderate continuous training in heart failure patients: A randomized study. Circulation 115(24):3086-3094, June 19, 2007.

30. Haram PM: Aerobic interval training vs. continuous moderate exercise in the metabolic syndrome of rats artificially selected for low aerobic capacity. Cardiovasc Res Dec 18, 2008; epub.

31. Thompson PD: Exercise and physical activity in the prevention and treatment of atherosclerotic cardiovascular disease: A statement from the Council on Clinical Cardiology. (Subcommittee on Exercise, Rehabilitation, and Prevention and the Council on Nutrition, Physical Activity, and Metabolism [Subcommittee on Physical Activity]). Circulation 107:3109-3116, 2003.

32. Lee KW, Lip GYH: Acute versus habitual exercise, thrombogenesis and exercise intensity. Thromb Haemost 91:416-419, 2004.

33. Piepoli MF: ExTra MATCH Collaborative. Exercise training meta-analysis of trials in patients with chronic heart failure. BMJ 328:189, 2004.

34. Pina IL: Exercise and heart failure: A statement from the American Heart Association Committee on exercise, rehabilitation, and prevention. Circulation 107(8):1210-1225, 2003.

35. Jones NL, Killian KJ: Exercise limitation in health and disease. NEJM 343(9):632-641, 2000.

36. American Academy of Orthopaedic Surgeons (AAOS): The Orthopaedics Update 2002 Web Conference, 2002. Available at www.aaos.org. Accessed January 22, 2009.

37. American Academy of Orthopaedic Surgeons: Beginning a weight training program. July 2007. Available at www.aaos.org. Accessed January 22, 2009.

38. American College of Sports Medicine (ACSM): Resource Manual for Guidelines for Exercise Testing and Prescription, 6th ed. Philadelphia, 2009.

Exercise Prescription

Before determining a plan of care including prescriptive exercise, the therapist must take into consideration the individual's health history, which requires documentation of the client's physical activity and exercise (type, frequency, intensity, and duration). This is a good opportunity to educate all clients about the importance of exercise as therapy for the many medical conditions discussed in this book. Counseling individuals on exercise has been shown effective in increasing physical activity and improving quality of life.[1]

Although many studies suggest that exercise provides various health benefits, the optimal type, frequency, intensity, and duration remain unknown for many specific conditions. These parameters may vary given the gender, age, personal and family health history, presence of variable comorbidities, current level of fitness, and so on. We envision that someday, as a result of careful research, it may be possible to outline specific and optimal dimensions for exercise taking these factors into consideration.

At the heart of the exercise prescription will be the physical therapist's knowledge of exercise physiology; energy metabolism; and cardiovascular, respiratory, musculoskeletal, and other systemic responses to exercise and training. Exercise prescription is a dynamic process requiring changes to maintain or advance training goals, to avoid overtraining, and provide optimal outcomes to targeted program (or health) goals.

The therapist begins with a single workout that is designed to reflect the goals through the type of exercise(s), and when appropriate the number of repetitions, sets used for each exercise, and intensity of each exercise. When exercise is new to an individual or the individual is starting again after an absence due to hospitalization, surgery, or some other reason, it may be necessary to encourage the person to go slow. The old adage of "No pain, no gain" is no longer valid. Rather, the new mantra is "No pain, big gains."

How Much Exercise Is Enough?

The key word is *moderate*. Moderate, painless, and enjoyable exercise is the best way to influence health and well-being. Clear health benefits have been shown with moderate exercise in lowering cholesterol, blood sugar, blood pressure, and body fat; slowing the effects of aging; reducing morbidity and mortality rates, and reducing the risk of many diseases.

For the overweight or obese individual, the importance of exercise should be stressed regardless of whether exercise results in weight loss. For anyone who is poorly motivated, overweight, or disabled, the idea that exercise must include an hour in the gym breathing hard and sweating should be dispelled and replaced with a program that will work (i.e., result in actual exercise) for the individual.

In fact, there is a broad spectrum of activities that contribute to health without being an intense workout at the gym. These activities fall into two categories: daily activities and recreational activities (e.g., gardening, dancing, yoga, washing the car by hand, golfing, dusting, raking the lawn, washing windows, sexual activity, snow shoveling, etc.) and are referred to as *cardiometabolic exercise* (CME). This new term emphasizes the idea that even activities at the lower end of intensity on a continuum still have major benefits on the cardiovascular and metabolic systems. Activities of all kinds are given CME points based on the activity itself, the pace (mild, moderate, heavy), and the duration in minutes (from 10 to 30).[2]

A good place for people of all ages to get started is the President's Council on Physical Fitness. There is no cost to participate. The Web site (www.presidentschallenge.org) allows visitors to create a personalized page to log in daily physical pursuits. Practical suggestions and guidelines are offered to show each age group ways to overcome a sedentary lifestyle or increase activity level.

The U.S. Centers for Disease Control and Prevention (CDC) and the American College of Sports Medicine (ACSM) recommend a minimum of 30 minutes of moderate-intensity physical activity most (if not all) days of the weeks (Box 2-1). People who do not exercise at all must be encouraged to begin with something much more manageable – like 1 to 3 minutes twice a day or a walk around the block after dinner. Sometimes just taking the stairs in public settings is an impressive goal. Even short 10-minute episodes of structured or nonstructured physical activity can be accumulated throughout the day adding up to 30 minutes has a proven benefit.[3]

For those who are already at this level and seeking greater fitness, Institute of Medicine (IOM) guidelines are for 60 minutes of moderate to vigorous physical activity most days to prevent weight gain and 60 to 90 minutes of daily physical activity to lose weight. A

Box 2-1 Current Recommendations	
American College of Sports Medicine	**Institute of Medicine**
30–40 minutes large-muscle-group activities 10,000 steps on a pedometer/day At least 5 days a week	60 minutes of moderate to vigorous physical activity to prevent weight gain 60–90 minutes of daily physical activity to lose weight A minimum of 30 minutes/day to reduce the risk of chronic disease

minimum of 30 minutes/day is still the target amount to reduce the risk of chronic disease. Moderate to vigorous exercise means the activity causes measurable changes in breathing and heart rate. How *much* change is part of the ongoing research to define. It is variable given a person's age, current level of fitness, and aerobic capacity. Different approaches have been taken based on Vo_2 max, rate of perceived exertion, target heart rate for sub-maximal to maximal aerobic conditioning, metabolic equivalents (METs), and so on.

Some researchers are approaching this from a slightly different perspective. One group of cardiologists has come up with a formula to determine the normal fitness level for women using METs to measure exercise capacity. For example, a 50-year-old woman should be able to reach 8.2 METs, the predicted exercise capacity for that age. The goal for a man the same age is 9.2 METs. Many exercise machines at health clubs include an analysis of METs, which usually means nothing to the person exercising. The results of this new research may help guide exercising individuals work at a level that will improve their fitness by giving them a goal to work toward and reaching their expected MET level.[4]

Using the Gulati model, *light-intensity* exercise is considered 2 to fewer than 4 METs for adults and 2 to fewer than 3 METs for older adults (age 55 and older). *Moderate-intensity* exercise is defined as 4 up to 6.4 METs for adults and 3 to fewer than 5 METs for older adults. Vigorous-intensity exercise is set from 6.5 METs and above for adults and 5 METs and more for older adults. Anything fewer than 2 METs does not contribute to habitual physical activity. Intensity scores can be calculated using the Short Questionnaire to Assess Health-Enhancing Physical Activity (SQUASH).[5]

Perhaps the most practical approach suggested utilizes a pedometer. Although pedometers are widely used as a physical activity monitoring tool, they are unable to measure activity intensity. San Diego State University researcher Simon Marshall has found a way to translate number of steps per minute into an exercise intensity. His practical rule-of-thumb for identifying "moderate intensity" comes from a study of healthy adult men and women recruited from the university. Using walking speed on a treadmill and calculating energy expended, he determined that a walking speed of at least 100 steps/minute could be defined as the lower limit of moderate intensity exercise in healthy adults. That translates into 3000 steps in 30 minutes. The reported range was 92 to 102 steps for men and 91 to 115 steps for women. Of course, this is to be considered a guideline that can be adapted for anyone based on the presence of any physical limitations. It can be used in combination with calculations for maximum heart rate (50% to 80% of 220 minus age).[6]

The simplest approach relies on the "talk test." If a person is breathing faster than normal but can still talk out loud, the person is exercising at a moderate intensity. Breathing with ease and carrying on a complete conversation would place the activity at the low-intensity level. Being breathless and unable to complete a sentence is gauged as high-intensity.

Progression of exercise is based more on common sense than on science at this point. The therapist evaluates each client's response(s) to the intervention and moves the client toward greater independence by matching the exercise program to the client's functional goals. In other words, when the client can do the exercise program easily, the frequency, intensity, and/or duration are changed to challenge the client further. This will certainly be addressed, but the research is not directed toward progression at this time.

Type (Mode), Frequency, Intensity, and Duration of Exercise

Components of the exercise prescription as outlined by the ACSM are *frequency*, *intensity*, *time* (duration), and *type* (mode) (FITT).[7] There is evidence that, as prescribed by a physician, people are more likely to comply when the prescription details the "dosage" as opposed to general advice to "exercise more."[8]

To date, the amount and intensity of exercise required for risk reduction for most conditions, especially heart disease, are not completely defined. Published studies suggest that if adults followed current physical activity guidelines for 30 minutes of daily, moderate activity, approximately 33% of deaths related to coronary heart disease, 25% of deaths related to strokes and osteoporosis, 20% of deaths related to colon cancer, hypertension, and type 2 diabetes, and 14% of deaths related to breast cancer could be prevented.[9]

Type or Mode of Exercise

Although exercise is often viewed as a single modality, it should be recognized that there is a great deal of variation among exercise programs and prescribed exercise protocols. Type of exercise encompasses short-term maximal exercise such as sprinting or climbing stairs; endurance exercise such as running, walking, or biking for long distances; and progressive exercise described as an increase in exercise until maximal capacity is reached.[10] There is also land-based versus pool therapy. None of these exercise types have the same effect on all people. Type or mode of exercise selected is determined by the individual's needs, goals, and ability level.

Despite recommendations for physical therapist–supervised exercise therapy for the management of numerous conditions, specific recommendations for type, frequency, and duration of the prescribed exercise are lacking in the literature. When there are so many different ways to set up exercise protocols, conducting research to investigate the effectiveness of exercise programs has many challenges. Performing systemic reviews does not always yield the necessary information. Many studies are of poor design and need improvement in methodology.[11]

Exercise training can be based on results of exercise testing, the individual's response to exercise, current medical status, risk factors, and personal goals. Exercise stress testing is not mandatory before beginning a moderate-intensity and moderately progressive exercise program, especially when supervised by a trained health-care professional such as the physical therapist. Support for this comes from a consensus group from the American Heart Association and the American College of Cardiology. Their recommendation comes from lack of well-established evidence on the usefulness and efficacy of routine exercise stress testing in healthy men older than 45 years and women older than 55 years.[12]

With many (but not all) diseases, illnesses, and conditions, there is a dose-gradient effect. In other words, as physical activity and exercise increase, the rates of disease decrease (e.g., diabetes, coronary artery disease, hypertension). In all cases, any activity is better than none. More vigorous exercise has greater benefits up to a point. There is also a boundary between healthy and unhealthy exercise. Developing optimal levels of exercise for individual conditions is the focus of many studies. There are stress responses to exercise that can be measured in all age groups. Research is being directed at finding the amount of exercise that stimulates the buildup of healthy cells and prevents excess cellular catabolism (breakdown) and degradation.

Some conditions require a different approach when it comes to type of exercise and what is considered the optimal frequency, intensity, and duration. For example, mild physical activity and exercise may boost immune function and keep the heart healthy, but they are not as effective in increasing bone density or preventing bone loss as specific resistance training.[13]

Duration of Exercise

Like any prescription, exercise prescription has a type and dosing frequency, intensity, and duration. As with frequency, duration is established based on individual short-term, intermediate, and long-term goals. These two parameters also depend on the individual's functional capacity as measured by METs. For people with a functional capacity less than 3 METs, exercise can begin with sessions lasting 5 to 10 minutes per session daily. As endurance increases, this is progressed upward to 3 to 5 METs in 15-minute sessions (twice daily) and to greater than 5 METs for 20 to 30 minutes three to five times/week.[14]

Training programs must expose individuals to enough training stimulus to challenge them physiologically but without overwhelming them with fatigue or other intolerable symptoms (e.g., muscle soreness, chest pain or angina pectoris, ventricular dysrhythmias, fatigue). This is one reason why a single formula for exercise prescription (i.e., one protocol used for everyone) detailing the exact frequency, intensity, and duration is not possible. Even though *frequency, intensity,* and *duration* are often used, the actual progression of training usually follows the order of duration, frequency, and intensity.

Frequency

How often should an individual exercise? Daily, of course, is the current advice for best practice. Duration may also guide frequency. For example, when starting out, some people may have to set a limit on how long they can exercise but try to fit two sessions in each day. As they build up their endurance, the duration can increase until they are able to complete a full 30-, 60-, or 90-minute workout. Others may have to remain with shorter duration and greater frequency. Smaller bouts of exercise added up still provide good benefits; sessions should be at least 10 minutes long to generate the same benefits as longer sessions.[15]

Exercise Intensity

Clients may need help establishing an intensity level. They may ask, "How hard should I push myself?" Intensity for aerobic exercise can be monitored using the Borg Scale for Rate of Perceived Exertion (RPE), with a baseline set for percent peak V_{O_2} of 40% to 50%. A peak heart rate of 60% RPE has been found to correlate with V_{O_2}. For example, Borg Scale ratings of 12 to 15 corresponding to light-moderate/heavy (on a scale from 6 to 20) correlates positively with 40% to 80% of peak V_{O_2}. This level of intensity is an acceptable training level for healthy subjects.[14]

Moderate-intensity exercise is needed to metabolize stored body fat and to modify physiologic functions that affect insulin, estrogen, androgen, prostaglandins, and immune function.[16] At the same time, the therapist should keep in mind that even when an individual does not meet the current recommendations for moderate-intensity physical activity requiring 3 METs or more, when intensity is perceived by the individual to be "moderate" to "strong or more intense," there is a heart-healthy response anyway.

Instead of applying this formula to every individual, fitness levels must be taken into consideration. If the client thinks the workout is tough enough, it probably is. In other words, perceived level of exertion is inversely related to the risk of developing heart disease.[17] Individuals should be encouraged to engage in physical activity at their own rate and level, gradually building intensity to receive maximal health benefits.

References

1. Elley CR: Effectiveness of counseling patients on physical activity in general practice: Cluster randomized controlled trial. BMJ 326:793, 2003.
2. Simon HB: The No Sweat Exercise Plan: Lose Weight, Get Healthy, and Live Longer. New York, McGraw-Hill, 2006.
3. Warburton DE: Prescribing exercise as preventive therapy. CMAJ 178(6):731-732, 2006.
4. Gulati M: The prognostic value of a nomogram for exercise capacity in women. NEJM 353(5):468-475, August 2005.
5. Wendel-Vos GC: Reproducibility and relative validity of the Short Questionnaire to Assess Health-Enhancing Physical Activity. J Clin Epidemiol 56:1163-1169, 2003.
6. Marshall S: Translating physical activity recommendations into a pedometer-based step goal. Am J Preventive Med 36(5):410-415, 2009.
7. American College of Sports Medicine: Resource Manual for Guidelines for Exercise Testing and Prescription, 6th ed. Philadelphia, 2009.
8. Grandes G: Effectiveness of physical activity advice and prescription by physicians in routine primary care: A cluster randomized trial. Arch Intern Med 169:694-701, 2009.
9. Warburton DE: Evidence-informed physical activity guidelines for Canadian adults. Can J Publ Health 98 Suppl 2:S16-68, 2007.
10. Jones NL, Killian KJ: Exercise limitation in health and disease. NEJM 343(9):632-641, 2000.
11. Helmhout PH: Exercise therapy and low back pain. Insights and proposals to improve the design, conduct, and reporting of clinical trials. Spine 33(16):1782-1788, 2008.
12. Gibbons RJ: ACC/AHA guidelines for exercise testing: A report of the American College of Cardiology/American Heart Association Task Force on Practice Guidelines. J Am Coll Cardiol 30:260-311, 1997.
13. Stewart KJ: Fitness, fatness, and activity as predictors of bone mineral density in older persons. J Int Med 252(5):381-388, 2002.
14. Heckman GA, McKelvie RS: Cardiovascular aging and exercise in healthy older adults. Clin J Sport Med 18(6):479-485, November 2008.
15. Haskell WL: American College of Sports Medicine and the American Heart Association: Physical activity and public health: Updated recommendations for adults. Med Sci Sports Exerc Special Communications 1423-1434, 2007.
16. Byers T: American Cancer Society guidelines on nutrition and physical activity for cancer prevention: Reducing the risk of cancer with healthy food choices and physical activity. Cancer J Clin 52:92-119, 2002.
17. Lee IM: Relative intensity of physical activity and risk of coronary heart disease. Circulation 107(8): 1110-1116, 2003.

Resources

Ashe MC, Khan KM: Exercise prescription. J Am Acad Orthop Surg 12(1):21-27, 2004.
Harvard Men's Health Watch: Exercise: A program you can live with, a special health report from Harvard Medical School. Boston, Harvard Health Publications, 2008. Available at www.health.harvard.edu. Accessed February 21, 2009.
Kraemer WJ, Ratamess NA: Fundamentals of resistance training: Progression and exercise prescription. Med Sci Sports Exerc 36(4):674-688, 2004.
Manson JE: Walking compared with vigorous exercise for the prevention of cardiovascular events in women. NEJM 347(10):716-725, 2002.

Chronic Illness and Disease

A sedentary lifestyle accounts for 250,000 or more premature deaths each year in the United States. About 10% of all deaths are attributed to inactivity, and almost 25% of all deaths are attributed to chronic illnesses. Fewer than 25% of all Americans get the exercise they need.[1]

Treating people with chronic disease accounts for approximately 75% of the over $2 trillion Americans spend on health care every year.[2] This may be explained by the 75 million adults in the United States age 50 years and older, many of whom have at least one chronic disease, such as arthritis, hypertension, or osteoporosis, that can be favorably affected by exercise. The role of exercise prescription in chronic disease has become a new focus in the shift to "exercise as medicine."[3]

Physical Activity for Chronic Disabling Diseases and Conditions

Exercise has been viewed most often as an activity for healthy people, not for the chronically ill. Physical activity is ranked as the leading health indicator in *Healthy People 2010*.[4,5] Endurance exercise reverses the cycle of deconditioning, weakness, and functional loss associated with many chronic disorders.[6]

There is a major research interest in examining the affect of physical activity and exercise on disability and other health outcomes, especially in older people. Studies such as the *Established Populations for Epidemiologic Studies of the Elderly (EPESE)* report data that show the number of years lived without disability depends on an active lifestyle. Even modest amounts of walking are associated with lower rates of disability onset. The EPESE is ongoing to evaluate the impact of exercise in preventing disability in nondisabled older adults.[7]

Supporting evidence continues to accumulate that physical activity and exercise reduce chronic disease risk directly through their impact on hormones and indirectly through their effect on weight control.[8] "Chronic disease management" is becoming a new term for rehabilitation in the treatment of chronic and disabling diseases, illnesses, conditions, and injuries.

Physical inactivity is associated with an increased risk for many chronic illnesses and disability, especially in the aging population. In people with chronic disease, exercise therapy is effective in increasing fitness and correcting some risk factors for the development of disease complications.[9,10] The numerous health benefits of regular physical activity have all been well documented. The accumulated knowledge is so extensive that the evidence must be translated into an implemented plan of action.[11]

Physical inactivity in an aging population is a major contributing factor to chronic illness and disability. Exercise has been proved to mitigate age-associated changes in the cardiovascular system.[12] Regular exercise, or sometimes just a modest increase in physical activity, has been shown to reduce muscle protein wasting associated with chronic diseases or conditions such as cancer, chronic real insufficiency, cachexia, sarcopenia, rheumatoid arthritis, osteoarthritis, and human immunodeficiency virus. The result can be increased endurance, strength, and even more independence in activities of daily living.[13,14]

Chronic diseases are divided by the American College of Sports Medicine into five major categories: cardiovascular and pulmonary, metabolic, immunologic/hematologic, orthopedic, and neuromuscular.[14] Research is under way to investigate the benefit and effectiveness of exercises for preventing chronic diseases in each category. As a result of the data collected so far, the federal government is starting to see the benefit of prevention and wellness interventions, especially related to chronic conditions. The Centers for Medicare and Medicaid Services (CMS) has announced a program under which it will match what states spend on disease-management programs for chronic conditions such as asthma, diabetes, and congestive heart failure.[15]

Current understanding of exercise prescription is limited for most chronic diseases.[3] Based on evidence, experience, and common sense, this text provides a summary of suggestions for specific training modes for a variety of medical diagnoses. It aims to be as current as possible as data become available. Guidelines for starting a basic exercise program are still relied upon when specifics were not available, always adjusting to accommodate any special considerations for the person or the disability.[16]

Exercise and the Immune System

There are known effects of exercise (beneficial and detrimental) on the number, functions, and characteristics of cells of the innate immune system.[17–20] Studies of moderate, vigorous, and strenuous exercise are increasingly showing how various levels of exercise intensity can alter immune function,[21,22] including exerting cancer-preventive effects. Exercise can reduce oxidative damage, enhance DNA repair systems, and improve intracellular protein repair systems. In other words, exercise is an immunomodulator.[23,24]

Overly vigorous exercise or overtraining (especially in a sedentary or unfit individual) can result in the formation of too many free radicals that can be damaging to the cells.[23] With the right type of exercise, proinflammatory mediators can be decreased in order to enhance macrophage and natural killer cell function and reduce low-grade chronic inflammation. This information is being used to attempt to reduce human susceptibility to infection and cancer.[25]

Aging and Exercise

Educating, promoting physical fitness, and preventing obesity, heart disease, type 2 diabetes, and other chronic health problems are all part of the role physical therapists have to play, starting with the pediatric population and encompassing all age groups across the lifespan.

The incidence of type 2 diabetes alone is rising dramatically in younger and younger people, including children. The benefits of physical fitness in the aging population are well-known in preventing falls and fractures, maintaining mobility and independence, and slowing functional decline. Exercise can increase oxygen saturation, reverse frailty, increase gait speed, reduce blood pressure, and thus enhance quality of life.[26]

Positive effects of physical activity and exercise on cognitive and brain function at the cellular, systems, and behavioral levels have been documented for all age groups, even for people in their 90s and 100s.[27–29] Even a moderate amount of daily physical activity can result in stronger bones, slower loss of muscle mass, improved balance, faster recovery from illness or injury, and reduced risk of many common diseases in older adults. Walking 4 hours per week has been shown to triple the 3-year survival rate for adults in their late 80s. Active octogenarians also report less depression and loneliness and a greater ability to perform daily tasks. Similar benefits have been shown in seniors ages 60 to 80 years.[30]

The results of many observational and interventional studies suggest that regular exercise (three or more times per week) is associated with a delay in onset of dementia and Alzheimer disease, further supporting its value for older adults. In fact, researchers say that even a modest amount of exercise can reduce a person's risk of dementia by about 40%.[31–35]

Short-term and long-term exercise may also release neurotransmitters (e.g., brain-derived neurotrophic factor [BDNF]), which promote cognitive function and brain health. Intensity of exercise has been shown to increase the benefit proportionally. This is an important finding given the fact that BDNF can pass through the blood-brain barrier in both directions. The intensity-dependent findings may aid in finding exercise prescriptions for maintaining or improving neurologic health.[36]

For the older adult (70 years and older), aerobic activity should remain in the functional range (as opposed to working at maximum aerobic capacity). This places the exercise in the submaximal aerobic range. Raising the heart rate above the resting level is the first goal; this must be done without exhausting the person's reserves for the remainder of the day's activities. Sometimes for the older, deconditioned adult, working on balance activities, strength training, and even flexibility can raise the heart rate into the submaximal zone. Monitoring vital signs is a good way to identify what level of activity the individual has reached.

The therapist should encourage daily exercise for at least 10 minutes (gradually building up tolerance from there), but advise all clients to take breaks from strength training. Give the muscles time to repair and recover, with a day's rest between 2 days of exercise. Fatigue, sore muscles, and a resting heart rate that is elevated by five or more beats over the normal morning rate indicate a person has not fully recovered from a workout and needs a break.[37] At the same time, do not let more than 36 hours pass between muscle-building activities to avoid losing the training effect.

Physically fit adults in the age range of 55 to 79 years have also shown less age-related brain tissue shrinkage in frontal, temporal, and parietal regions of the brain as compared with less active adults the same ages.[38] Aerobic fitness training can combat this effect by enhancing the cognitive vitality of healthy but sedentary older adults.[30] This same study[38] also found that whereas small amounts of exercise are beneficial in many physiologic ways, exercising less than 30 minutes per session has very little impact on cognitive function.[39] The activity can be as simple as brisk walking. With a gradual increase in activity from 30 to 45 minutes, an 11% improvement in decision making performed while carrying out a variety of tasks has been demonstrated.

Mental Health and Cognitive Function

Exercise has been shown to improve a sense of well-being, reduce anxiety, enhance problem solving, and is often prescribed in the treatment of anxiety and depressive (mood) disorders.[40] Not everyone will tolerate the exercise prescriptions provided in this text, given individual age, mental competency, comorbidities, and other compromising conditions. Aerobic exercise prompts the release of endorphins, serotonin, and other mood-lifting hormones. The result is stress relief, increased sense of well-being, and better sleep patterns.[41] Physical activity enhances cognitive and brain function and protects against cognitive decline and the development of neurodegenerative diseases.[42,43]

Observational studies suggest that physically active adults are less likely to experience cognitive decline and dementia compared with less sedentary groups.[33] Regular endurance exercise can improve cognition in older adults who are sedentary.[39,44,45] Cognitively impaired older adults with dementia should be involved in exercise rehabilitation; positive outcomes are equal to those of matched controls with normal cognitive function who exercise.[46] There is a strong biologic basis for the role of aerobic fitness in maintaining and enhancing central nervous system health and cognitive functioning in older adults.

Animal studies have shown that exercise reduces cellular damage in brain cells from oxidation, which is believed to be associated with memory loss and possibly Alzheimer disease in humans. Brain cells in rats that engaged in regular moderate exercise had healthier molecular fats and DNA samples than rats that did not exercise. The results indicate that lifelong exercise attenuates multiple molecular markers of age-related oxidative damage in the cerebellum. In addition, modest exercise initiated late in life had a beneficial effect on lipid oxidation and motor function.[47]

Aerobic-based exercise training and resistance training have been shown to have a protective role in lowering the risk of cognitive impairment and dementia. Resistance training may prevent cognitive decline via mechanisms involving IGF-1 and homocysteine.[48] Aerobic fitness (higher fitness levels) has been linked with a larger brain hippocampus, which translates to better memory function.[49]

Unlike medication, physical activity has health benefits that are not confined to cognitive function. Physical activity and exercise reduce physical disability, depression, and the incidence of falls as well as increase quality of life and improve cardiovascular function. The beneficial effects of physical activity are sustained over time.[33]

High-quality studies are lacking in evidence as to the specific type of exercise best suited to maintain or improve cognitive control. More high-quality trials are needed to assess the effects of different types of exercise on cognitive function in older adults with and without cognitive decline.[50] Feasibility studies and systematic reviews of exercise on cognition in older adults with mild cognitive impairment support the idea that regular moderate-intensity walking improves aerobic fitness. Small but significant improvements were observed in program attendance and memory with improved aerobic fitness.[50,51]

Guidelines set out so far for aerobic, resistance, and balance training for healthy older adults have been published, based on recommendations from the American Heart Association and the American College of Sports Medicine. The American Academy of Orthopaedic Surgeons suggests that older athletes engage in low-impact endurance activities and sports rather than high-impact activities.[52–54]

References

1. Harvard Men's Health Watch: Exercise: A program you can live with, a special health report from Harvard Medical School. Boston, Harvard Health Publications, 2008. Available at www.health.harvard.edu. Accessed December 12, 2009.
2. Royall RS, Rear Admiral: US Deputy Assistant Secretary for Health in the US Department of Health and Human Services. PTs: First responders: Keynote address. PT 2007: Annual conference and exposition of the American Physical Therapy Association, Denver, CO, June 2007.
3. Moore GE: The role of exercise prescription in chronic disease. Br J Sports Med 38:6-7, 2004.
4. U.S. Department of Health and Human Services. Physical activity and health: A report of the Surgeon General. U.S. Department of Health and Human Services, Centers for Disease Control and Prevention, National Center for Chronic Disease Prevention and Health Promotion, Atlanta, GA, 1996.
5. U.S. Department of Health and Human Services. Healthy People 2010: Understanding and improving health, 2nd ed. U.S. Government Printing Office, Washington, DC, 2000.
6. Iverson MD: Enhancing function in older adults with chronic low back pain: A pilot study of endurance training. Arch Phys Med Rehabil 84(9):1324-1331, 2003.
7. Guralnik JM: Established populations for epidemiologic studies of the elderly (EPESE). National Institute on Aging, 2005. Available at www.grc.nia.nih.gov/brances/ledb/jguralnik.htm. Accessed January 7, 2009.
8. Eyre H: Preventing cancer, cardiovascular disease, and diabetes: A common agenda for the American Cancer Society, the American Diabetes Association, and the American Heart Association. Am Cancer J Clin 54:190-207, 2004.
9. Kujala UM: Evidence for exercise therapy in the treatment of chronic disease based on at least three randomized controlled trials: Summary of published systematic reviews. Scand J Med Sci Sports 14: 339-345, 2004.
10. Kujala UM: Benefits of exercise therapy for chronic diseases. Br J Sports Med 40(1):3-4, 2006.
11. Pedersen BK, Saltin B: Evidence for prescribing exercise as therapy in chronic disease. Scand J Med Sci Sports 16(Suppl 1):3-63, 2006.
12. Heckman GA, McKelvie RS: Cardiovascular aging and exercise in healthy older adults. Clin J Sports Med 18(6):479-485, November 2008.
13. Zinna EM: Exercise treatment to counteract protein wasting of chronic disease. Curr Opin Nutr Metab Care 6(1):87-93, 2003.
14. Durstine JL: ACSM's exercise management for persons with chronic diseases and disabilities, 2nd ed. Champaign, IL, 2002.
15. Centers for Medicare and Medicaid Services (CMS): CMS offers funds for Medicaid disease management. http://www.cms.hhs.gov/. Posted February 27, 2004. Accessed January 19, 2009.
16. Durstine JL: Physical activity for the chronically ill and disabled. Sports Med 30(3):207-219, 2000.
17. Woods JA, Davis JM, Smith JA: Exercise and cellular innate immune function. Med Sci Sports Exerc 31(1):57-66, 1999.
18. Wang JS: Exercise affects platelet-impeded antitumor cytotoxicity of natural killer cell. Med Sci Sports Exerc 41(1):115-122, 2009.

19. Chen YW: Exercise affects platelet-promoted tumor cell adhesion and invasion to endothelium. Eur J Appl Physiol 105(3):393-401, 2009.
20. Matthews CE: Moderate to vigorous physical activity and risk of upper-respiratory tract infection. Med Sci Sports Exerc 34(8):1242-1248, 2002.
21. Goodman CC, Kapasi ZF: The effect of exercise on the immune system. Rehabil Oncol 20(1):13-26, 2002.
22. Kapasi ZF: Effect of duration of a moderate exercise program on primary and secondary immune responses. Phys Ther 83(7):638-647, 2003.
23. Rogers CJ: Physical activity and cancer prevention: Pathways and targets for intervention. Sports Med 38(4):271-296, 2008.
24. Senchina DS, Kohut ML: Immunological outcomes of exercise in older adults. Clin Intervent Aging 2(1): 3-16, 2007.
25. Mitchell T: Move yourself: The Cooper Clinic medical director's guide to all the healing benefits of exercise (even a little!). Hoboken, NJ, John Wiley & Sons, 2008.
26. Moffat M: Physical fitness: Promoting health and wellness in all patient/client populations. Plenary session. Annual Conference and Exposition of the American Physical Therapy Association, June 2007, Denver, CO.
27. Hillman CH: Be smart, exercise your heart: Exercise effects on brain and cognition. Natl Rev Neurosci 9(1):58-65, 2008.
28. Ljubuncic P: Evidence-based roads to the promotion of health in old age. J Nutr Health Aging 12(2): 139-143, 2008.
29. Ozaki A: The Japanese centenarian study: Autonomy was associated with health practices as well as physical status. J Am Geriatr Soc 55(1):95-101, 2007.
30. Stessman J: Physical activity, function, and longevity among the very old. Arch Intern Med 169(16): 1476-1483, 2009.
31. Larson EB: Exercise is associated with reduced risk for incident dementia among persons 65 years of age and older. Ann Intern Med 144(2):73-81, 2006.
32. Larson EB: Physical activity for older adults at risk for Alzheimer's disease. JAMA 300(9):1077-1099, 2008. [See also http://www.medscape.com/viewarticle/521660?src=mp]
33. Lautenschlager NT: Effect of physical activity on cognitive function in older adults at risk for Alzheimer's disease: A randomized trial. JAMA 300(9):1027-1037, 2008.
34. Ma Q: Beneficial effects of moderate voluntary physical exercise and its biological mechanisms on brain health. Neurosci Bull 24(4):265-270, 2008.
35. Rolland Y: Physical activity and Alzheimer's disease: From prevention to therapeutic perspectives. J Am Med Dir Assoc 9(6):390-405, 2008.
36. Ferris L: The effect of acute exercise on serum brain-derived neurotrophic factor levels and cognitive function. Med Sci Sports Exerc 39(4):728-734, 2007.
37. DiNubile NA: How much exercise is too much? AAOS Bulletin 2008. Available at www.aaos.org. Accessed January 21, 2009.
38. Colcombe S: Aerobic fitness reduces brain tissue loss in aging humans. J Gerontol 58:M176-M180, 2003.
39. Colombe S, Kramer AF: Fitness effects on the cognitive function of older adults: A meta-analytic study. Psychol Sci 14(2):125-130, 2003.
40. Callaghan P: Exercise: A neglected intervention in mental health care? J Psychiatr Mental Health Nurse 11(4):476-483, 2004.
41. Lee I-Min: Exercise: A program you can live with: A special report from Harvard Medical School. Boston, Harvard University Press, 2003.
42. Kramer AF, Erickson KI: Capitalizing on cortical plasticity: Influence of physical activity on cognition and brain function. Trends Cognitive Sci 11(8):342-348, 2008.
43. Yaffe K: A prospective study of physical activity and cognitive decline in elderly women. Arch Intern Med 161:1703-1708, 2001.
44. Colcombe SJ: Aerobic exercise training increases brain volume in aging adults. J Gerontol A Biol Sci Med Sci 61(11):1166-1170, 2006.
45. Hillman CH: Be smart, exercise your heart: Exercise effects on brain and cognition. Nature Rev Neurosci 9:58-65, 2008.
46. Heyn PC: Endurance and strength training outcomes on cognitively impaired and cognitively intact older adults: A meta-analysis. J Nutr Health Aging 12(6):401-409, 2008.
47. Cui L: Comparison of lifelong and late life exercise on oxidation stress in the cerebellum. Neurobiol Aging 30(6):903-909, 2009.
48. Liu-Ambrose T, Donaldson M: Exercise and cognition in older adults: Is there a role for resistance training programs? Br J Sports Med Nov. 19, 2008.

49. Erickson KI: Aerobic fitness is associated with hippocampal volume in elderly humans. Hippocampus 19(10):1030-1039, 2009.
50. Van Uffelen JG: The effects of exercise on cognition in older adults with and without cognitive decline: A systematic review. Clin J Sports Med 18(6):486-500, November 2008.
51. Chin A, Paw MJ: The functional effects of physical exercise training in frail older people: A systematic review. Sports Med 38(9):781-793, 2008.
52. American College of Sports Medicine. ACSM's Guidelines for Exercise Testing and Prescription, 7th ed. Philadelphia, Lippincott, Williams & Wilkins, 2005.
53. Lauer M: Exercise testing in asymptomatic adults: A statement for professionals from the American Heart Association. Circulation 112:771-776, 2005.
54. American Academy of Orthopaedic Surgeons (AAOS): Older athletes exercising their options. JOMM 22(11):558-559, 2005.

Conditions

The following section contains information about prescribing exercise for clients with specific medical conditions. Each chapter includes information about the pathophysiology of the condition and how the condition results in an endurance impairment or limits the clients' physical activities. The chapter then provides key information for examining the clients and how to take baseline measurements of fitness levels. An outline of recommended exercise parameters and specific information for how exercise should progress for these clients completes each chapter. This information assumes the reader has some background in assessing fitness levels and has some experience in prescribing appropriate exercise parameters. Finally, a short list of references demonstrates the best evidence for exercise prescriptions for that particular condition and provides readily available resources of in-depth information about these exercise prescriptions. References listed represent only a small portion of the available literature; we attempted to condense and summarize the best evidence for each condition.

LIST OF CONDITIONS

ACQUIRED IMMUNE DEFICIENCY SYNDROME (AIDS)

Overview of AIDS

This condition is a suppression of the immune system from a progressive loss of cell-mediated and humoral immunity. The condition begins with the infection by the human immunodeficiency retrovirus (HIV) leading to the loss of T4-cell lymphocytes. A state of immunodeficiency results in clients being susceptible to infections, cancers, and other conditions. Clients will be on highly active antiretroviral therapies to suppress the effects of the HIV. Clients may have fatigue from secondary infections and other conditions that limit their daily activities, thus leading to deconditioning.[1,2] The implementation of a prescribed exercise program will reverse the effects of deconditioning without adversely affecting the clients' immune deficiency.[3]

Comorbidities to Consider

• Clients who develop painful peripheral neuropathies, arthritic conditions, and myopathies may need to limit activities to control symptoms.

Client Examination

Keys to Examination of Clients

• Ask the clients about their current level of lymphocytes; a CD4 lymphocyte count below 500/mm^3 indicates immune deficiency.
• Discuss with the clients what type of testing and treatment are being received for secondary conditions.

Recommended Baseline Testing of Fitness Levels

• Cardiovascular fitness can be assessed with submaximal testing via treadmill, cycle ergometer, or walking tests.
• Muscle strength can be determined through free or machine weights using one-repetition or ten-repetition maximum testing.
• An assessment of the clients' level of anxiety or depression can be useful to determine the psychological effects of an exercise program.[3,4]

Exercise Prescription

Type: Combination of aerobic and resistive exercise
Intensity: 60%–75% of maximum heart rate[3,5]
Duration: Start at 20 minutes
Frequency: Three to five sessions per week.

Getting Started

Carefully choose the initial exercise parameters, and instruct your clients to avoid overexertion as they will need to avoid excessive fatigue to maintain a healthy immune system. Clients suffering bouts of depression, excessive anxiety, or poor sleep quality should maintain some level of exercise but may need to decrease the intensity of their exercise program.[6] Clients should maintain their exercise program for at least 6 months to attain age-normal levels of endurance and cardiovascular fitness. Clients should benefit from the physical and psychologic effects of their exercise program.[3,4] When clients have progressed to a consistent exercise program, add resistive exercises for major muscle groups. Resistive exercises can be performed with intensities at 60% of maximum with 3 sets of 10 repetitions and a rest period of 1 to 2 minutes between sets.[3,7,8] Clients with AIDS may be able to progress their exercise programs to include moderate- and high-intensity aerobic and recreational activities.[3]

References

1. Hand GA, Phillips KD, Dudgeon WD, et al. Moderate intensity exercise training reverses functional aerobic impairment in HIV-infected individuals. AIDS Care 20(9):1066-1074, 2008.
2. Cade WT, Peralta L, Keyser RE. Aerobic exercise dysfunction in human immunodeficiency virus: A potential link to physical disability. Phys Ther 84(7):644-654, 2004.
3. Ciccolo JT, Esbelle EM, Bartholomew JB. The benefits of exercise training for quality of life in HIV/AIDS in the post-HAART era. Sports Med 34(8):487-499, 2004.
4. Dudgeon WD, Phillips KD, Bopp CM, et al. Physiological and psychological effects of exercise interventions in HIV disease. AIDS Patient Care STDS 18(2):81-98, 2004.
5. Nixon S, O'Brien K, Grazier R, et al. Aerobic exercise interventions for adults living with HIV/AIDS. Cochrane Database Syst Rev 2:CD001796, 2005.
6. Phillips KD, Sowell RL, Rojas M, et al. Physiological and psychological correlates of fatigue in HIV disease. Biol Res Nurs 6(1):59-74, 2004.
7. Fillipas S, Oldmeadow LB, Bailey MJ, et al. A six-month, supervised, aerobic and resistance exercise program improves self-efficacy in people with human immunodeficiency virus: A randomised controlled trial. Austr J Phys 52:185-190, 2006.
8. O'Brien K, Nixon S, Glazier R, et al. Progressive resistive exercise interventions for adults living with HIV/AIDS. AIDS Care 20(6):631-653, July 2008.

ANEMIA

Overview of Anemia

This condition is due to the decreased quantity or quality of red blood cells and results in a decline in the capacity of the blood to carry oxygen. Anemia is considered a sign of any disorder that affects the production, normal destruction, or loss of red blood cells. Anemia is defined by hemoglobin levels of less than 12 g/100 dL for women and less than 14 g/100 dL for men. Clients may experience anemia as a temporary result of an injury or disease process or may need ongoing treatments to maintain an adequate supply of oxygen in the blood stream. Clients with anemia may experience fatigue, dyspnea, and weakness, which will limit their daily activities.

Comorbidities to Consider

- Clients undergoing treatment for diseases that create anemia, such as cancers and bone marrow disorders, may also have limited mobility due to these diseases.
- A long-term reduction in activities can lead to secondary deconditioning effects for the cardiovascular and neuromusculoskeletal systems.

Client Examination

Keys to Examination of Clients

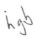

- Clients with anemia will be assessed by complete blood counts, counts of red blood cell indices, and levels of serum iron, serum ferritin, and vitamin B_{12}.

Recommended Baseline Testing of Fitness Levels

- Clients can be assessed for their tolerance to exercise activities with walking or cycle ergometer tests.[1] Testing should be performed with close monitoring of vital signs and with slow progression of exercise intensities.
- Clients may also need to be assessed for balance and coordination by standing and walking activities, as some chronic conditions produce peripheral neuropathies.

Exercise Prescription

Type: Walking, cycling, arm ergometer, and acquatic activities
Intensity: Low levels
Duration: Short durations, 10–20-minute bouts with rest periods
Frequency: Daily as tolerated

Getting Started

Walking activities will be the most common form of exercise for clients with severe debilitation due to primary conditions that create anemia.[1] Clients may choose aquatic exercise program when taking safety precautions. Clients with anemia will need close and ongoing monitoring of their heart rate, oxygen saturation levels, and dyspnea levels during exercise sessions. Exercise intensities can be self-assessed by perceived exertion levels or by taking heart rate levels during the exercise program. Monitoring of oxygen saturation and heart rate will help determine when clients are exercising in a state of decreased blood oxygen. The parameters of exercise will need to be appropriate for the clients' primary or secondary condition that has created their anemia.[2,3] Daily levels of fatigue should be assessed to prescribe an appropriate level of exercise based on clients' progression or deterioration from their primary condition.[4] Clients can be progressed to independent exercise programs to increase their functional capacities and improve their cardiovascular health.

References

1. Dean E. Oxygen transport deficits in systemic disease and implications for physical therapy. Phys Ther 77(2):187-202, 1997.
2. Watson T, Mock V. Exercise as an intervention for cancer-related fatigue. Phys Ther 84(8):736-743, 2004.
3. Durstine JL, Painter P, Franklin BA, et al. Physical activity for the chronically ill and disabled. Sports Med 30(3):207-219, Sep 2000.
4. Drouin JS, Young TJ, Beeler J, et al. Random control clinical trial on the effects of aerobic exercise training on erythrocyte levels during radiation treatment for breast cancer. Cancer 107(10):2490-2495, Nov 15, 2006.

ANKYLOSING SPONDYLITIS

Overview of Ankylosing Spondylitis

This systemic inflammatory condition primarily affects the sacroiliac joints and joints of the spine and can also affect peripheral joints. The condition leads to fibrosis and ossification of the involved articulations. The cause of the condition is unknown, although it may have environmental and genetic origins. This condition is usually initiated by an insidious onset of low back or hip pain and stiffness. Severe complications, including spinal stenosis and vertebral fractures, that limit mobility can occur. Individuals with this condition will have limited mobility due to joint stiffness that is particularly severe in the morning. Pain and related fatigue symptoms will limit their ability to initiate exercise and recreational activities.

Comorbidities to Consider

* Advanced ankylosing spondylitis limits chest wall mobility and leads to respiratory muscle fatigue that will significantly limit exercise tolerance.[1]

Client Examination

Keys to Examination of Clients

* This condition is not easily identifiable during its early stages.
* Consider recommending radiographs, which may show signs of sacroiliitis and inflammation in the spinal articulations.
* Laboratory tests for the HLA-B27 antigen may assist in identifying this condition.
* Assess clients' posture, chest expansion, and range of motion of the spine and extremities to determine a baseline for these impairments.

Recommended Baseline Testing of Fitness Levels

* Exercise tolerance can be assessed by walking or cycle ergometer tests.
* The Bath Ankylosing Spondylitis Disease Activity Index can be used as a baseline for the patient's symptoms and activity level.[2]

Exercise Prescription

Type: Walking, biking, postural and pulmonary exercises, and stretching activities[3-5]
Intensity: Low levels to start, aerobic activities at 50%–60% of maximum heart rate[3]
Duration: Up to 50 minutes of combined activities
Frequency: Three times per week

Getting Started

Clients with this condition have limited spinal mobility and abnormal spinal postures, which increases their risk for sustaining vertebral fractures. Start clients in the exercise program with a warm-up period of stretching and stepping or walking activities. Take the time to individually teach these clients exercises to address their spinal posture, chest wall mobility, and muscle tightness to ensure proper form and tolerance. Avoid excessive exercise intensities or stretching procedures that may worsen the inflammatory process. Exercises that potentially require excessive joint motion, such as rowing or an elliptical trainer, should be avoided when beginning an exercise program. Aquatic therapies have also been recommended for clients with this condition. Supervised and group exercise programs are recommended for clients beginning a program or for those with recent exacerbation of symptoms.[6,7] Clients should be encouraged to progress to an independent exercise program to maintain their fitness and mobility.[6]

References

1. Fisher LR, Cawley MI, Holgate ST. Relation between chest expansion, pulmonary function, and exercise tolerance in patients with ankylosing spondylitis. Ann Rheum Dis 49(11):921-925, 1990.
2. Bath Ankylosing Spondylitis Disease Activity Index. http://www.basdai.com/BASDAI.php. Accessed November 24, 2009.
3. Ince G, Sarpel T, Durgen B. Effects of a multimodal exercise program for people with ankylosing spondylitis. Phys Ther 86(7):924-935, 2006.
4. Fernández-de-Las-Peñas C, Alonso-Blanco C, Alguacil-Diego IM, et al. One-year follow-up of two exercise interventions for the management of patients with ankylosing spondylitis: A randomized controlled trial. Am J Phys Med Rehabil 85(7):559-567, 2006.
5. National Ankylosing Spondylitis Association's Guidebook for Patients. http://www.nass.co.uk/public/zips/NassBook.pdf. Accessed September 2, 2009.
6. Dagfinrud H, Kvien TK, Hagen KB. Physiotherapy interventions for ankylosing spondylitis. Cochrane Database Syst Rev 1:CD002822, 2008.
7. Dougados M, Dijkmans B, Khan M. Conventional treatments for ankylosing spondylitis. Ann Rheum Dis Suppl 3:40-50, Dec 2002.

ANXIETY DISORDERS

Overview of Anxiety Disorders

These disorders are emotional states of apprehension and fear that create physiologic arousal responses mediated through the sympathetic system. These disorders include adjustment disorders, post-traumatic stress disorder, obsessive-compulsive disorders, and general anxiety disorder. Individuals with these disorders can exhibit numerous abnormal signs and symptoms that are also associated with physical activities. Clients with these conditions typically avoid exercise activities, as normal responses to exercise can be interpreted as an increase in their state of anxiety.[1] Clients with anxiety disorders benefit from behavioral therapies, medications, and exercise programs to manage their anxiety levels.[1,2]

Concurrent Symptoms That May Occur With Anxiety Disorders

Increase respiration rate	Elevated heart rate
Elevated blood pressure	Increased muscle tension
Sweating	Irritability
Hyperalertness	Dizziness

Comorbidities to Consider

- Clients with heart disease and pulmonary conditions may have significant deconditioning that limits their daily activities.

Client Examination

Keys to Examination of Clients

- Screen your clients for heart disease and any physical limitations before they begin an exercise program.
- Perform testing and the beginning of an exercise program in a controlled environment to limit the effects on their level of anxiety.
- Discuss with your clients the benefit of exercise for controlling their levels of anxiety and their readiness to begin an exercise program.

Recommended Baseline Testing of Fitness Levels

- Assess aerobic capacity with activities with which the client is familiar, such as walking, treadmill walking, or cycle ergometry testing.
- Vital signs need to be assessed before and during exercise to ensure that changes are due to normal physiologic responses.
- Clients should be screened for their overall mobility and if any comorbidities will limit their exercise activities.

Exercise Prescription

Type: Walking, biking, running, weight lifting
Intensity: Moderate, progressing to high levels, 70%-90% of maximum heart rate[3-6]
Duration: At least 20 minutes per day
Frequency: 5–7 days per week

Getting Started

Clients with anxiety disorders benefit the most from higher intensity exercise performed 5 to 7 days per week for 30 to 60 minutes.[3,5] Add resistance training into the exercise program using parameters that promote aerobic capacity, and maintain a regular exercise program. Encourage these clients to adopt a variety of activities that promote aerobic fitness to maintain their fitness levels and to manage their anxiety levels. Clients who successfully manage their anxiety disorders may be encouraged to participate in competitive endurance events. Anticipate that clients may need to participate in regular aerobic activities for up to 10 weeks before experiencing significant reduction in their anxiety levels.[1,2]

References

1. Phongsavan P, Merom D, Wagner R, et al. Process evaluation in an intervention designed to promote physical activity among adults with anxiety disorders: Evidence of acceptability and adherence. Health Promotion J Austr 19(2):137-143, 2008.
2. Petruzzello SJ, Landers DM, Hatfield BD, et al. A meta-analysis on the anxiety-reducing effects of acute and chronic exercise: Outcomes and mechanisms. Sports Med 11(3):143-182, 1991.
3. Wipfli BM, Rethorst CD, Landers DM. The anxiolytic effects of exercise: A meta-analysis of randomized trials and dose-response analysis. J Sport Exerc Psychol 30(4):392-410, 2008.
4. Merom D, Phongsavan P, Wagner R, et al. Promoting walking as an adjunct intervention to group cognitive behavioral therapy for anxiety disorders: A pilot group randomized trial. J Anxiety Disord 22(6):959-968, 2008.
5. Dunn AL, Trivedi MH, O'Neal HA. Physical activity dose-response effects on outcomes of depression and anxiety. Med Sci Sports Exerc 33(6 Suppl):S587-S597, 2001.
6. Broman-Fulks JJ, Storey KM. Evaluation of a brief aerobic exercise intervention for high anxiety sensitivity. Anxiety Stress Coping 21(2):117-128, 2008.

ASTHMA

Overview of Asthma

This is a chronic inflammatory disease, which produces a reversible obstructive lung condition during exacerbation episodes. Asthma can be triggered by numerous environmental causes, which include exercise activities. Inflammation of airways produces edema, mucous production, and smooth muscle spasms that obstruct the airway, thus making breathing difficult. Bronchospasms produce wheezing, with prolonged expirations, a nonproductive cough, and tachypnea. Progression of the disease can lead to permanent changes in the airway similar to those of other chronic obstructive pulmonary diseases.[1] Individuals with this condition may experience exercise-induced asthma, especially in cold weather conditions. These attacks can be unpredictable and may cause the individual to limit exercise activities to avoid these episodes. Clients with asthma can improve their aerobic fitness and breathing reserve without increasing the occurrence of asthma and may improve their ability to recover from an asthmatic episode.[2,3]

Comorbidities to Consider

- Clients who are obese have a greater risk for developing asthma. The effects of obesity make asthma difficult to control.

Client Examination

Keys to Examination of Clients

- Ask clients if they have had pulmonary function studies, arterial blood gas analysis, and chest radiographs to assess the severity of their disease.
- Assess for breathing patterns, proper use of inhaler medication, and postures during exercise activities.[4]
- Counsel clients who smoke or use tobacco on the effects of smoke and nicotine on their medical condition.
- Discuss with younger clients their beliefs about physical activities and their asthma. Many adolescents avoid activities that could bring on asthmatic episodes to avoid appearing different from their peers and as an excuse for sedentary behaviors.[5,6]

Recommended Baseline Testing of Fitness Levels

- Choose aerobic tests of walking, running, or cycling will allow for baseline measurements of aerobic capacity, ventilation measures, and airway tolerance of exercise activities.
- Document the types of activities and the environmental triggers that have caused the onset of their asthmatic episodes to determine a baseline for their tolerance to activities.

Exercise Prescription

Type: A variety of recreational and competitive activities
Intensity: 50% of peak oxygen uptake or at limits tolerated by symptoms[7]
Duration: 20–30 minutes
Frequency: Three to five times per week

Getting Started

Clients with severe forms of asthma will need to modify their participation to avoid asthmatic episodes.[2] Swimming has been considered the least likely activity to promote an asthmatic episode, due to the benefits of breathing warm, humid air.[8] Clients should learn how to use perceived exertion, breathlessness levels, and other symptoms to control their level of exercise intensity to avoid developing an asthmatic episode. Clients need to recognize when they begin to breathe more through their mouth in response to the increased intensity or duration of their activity.[2] Clients need to avoid environmental conditions of breathing cold, dry air and need to use a scarf or mask to warm the air. Clients with severe symptoms should start exercise sessions with long warm-up periods, use a bronchodilator medication 20 to 30 minutes before starting exercise, and have their bronchodilators available during exercise sessions. Clients participating in sports activities should be encouraged to have rest periods during their practices and competitions. Clients should learn how to control their asthmatic symptoms through education and medication in order to participate in a variety of activities to maintain their fitness and sustain a high quality of living.

References

1. Asthma and Allergy Foundation of America. http://www.aafa.org/display.cfm?id=4&sub=79&cont=432. Accessed November 24, 2009.
2. Welsh L, Kemp JG, Roberts R. Effects of physical conditioning on children and adolescents with asthma. Sports Med 35(2):127-141, 2005.
3. Ram FS, Robinson SM, Black PN, et al. Physical training for asthma. Cochrane Database Syst Rev 19(4):CD001116, 2005.
4. Lavorini F, Magnan A, Dubus JC, et al. Effect of incorrect use of dry powder inhalers on management of patients with asthma and COPD. Respir Med 102(4):593-604, 2008.
5. Callery P, Milnes L, Veduyn C, et al. Qualitative study of young people's and parents' beliefs about childhood asthma. Br J Gen Pract 53(488):185-190, 2003.
6. Williams B, Powell A, Hoskins G, et al. Exploring and explaining low participation in physical activity among children and young people with asthma: A review. BMC Fam Pract 9:40, 2008
7. Lucas SR, Platts-Mills T. Physical activity and exercise in asthma: Relevance to etiology and treatment. J Allergy Clin Immunol. 115(5):928-934, 2005.
8. Rosimini C. Benefits of swim training for children and adolescents with asthma. J Am Acad Nurse Pract 15(6):247-252, 2003.

BONE MARROW TRANSPLANT

Overview of Bone Marrow Transplant

A transplant of hematopoietic stem cells from bone marrow, peripheral blood, or umbilical cord blood into a client's bone marrow is a life-saving procedure. Clients typically have a type of cancer that requires chemotherapy or radiation that destroys the bone marrow in order to stop the progression of their disease. The bone marrow is repopulated with healthy stem cells that can differentiate into mature blood cells. The hematopoietic stem cells can be from an allogeneic donor, usually a close relative, or from the person's own (autologous) blood. Clients undergoing this procedure may have numerous complications that will require hospitalization and involvement of many health-care providers. This procedure places the client under a great amount of physical, emotional, and psychosocial stress.[1] Clients are deconditioned due to significant declines in function and independence resulting from treatment of their disease process and the transplant procedure.[2] Exercise interventions after hematopoietic stem cell transplantation have many potential benefits for the client.[1]

Potential Effects of an Exercise Program

Improved endurance
Decreased fatigue levels
Improved body composition

Improved strength
Improved quality of life
Improved mood states

Comorbidities to Consider

- Clients may have hemorrhagic complications and compromised immunity for a long period after their transplant.

Client Examination

Keys to Examination of Clients

- Determine clients' readiness for activities by assessing the results of blood tests, especially platelet counts. Determine if clients need further assessments of their cardiac and pulmonary function.
- Assess clients' vital signs and levels of fatigue to maintain a proper level of exercise intensity and endurance.
- Look for early signs of transplant rejection, which include dyspnea, chest pain, irregular heart rate, and increasing fatigue, all of which may be exhibited during an exercise session.
- Post-transplant pain syndromes with mouth sores, diarrhea, nausea, and fatigue can limit exercise adherence.
- Opioid (narcotic) medications used to treat pain can also reduce the motivation to maintain an exercise program.[3]

Recommended Baseline Testing of Fitness Levels

- Aerobic fitness can be assessed by walking or cycle ergometry testing.
- Muscle strength is best assessed by isometric or isotonic movements with larger muscle groups in the upper and lower extremities, along with grip strength.[4]
- Assess clients' overall mobility and muscle flexibility if clients have been hospitalized for an extended period.
- Assess fatigue levels and physical function levels throughout the course of treatment.[1]

Exercise Prescription

Type: Treadmill walking, cycle ergometry
Intensity: Start at 60%–70% of predicted maximum heart rate
Duration: 10–20 minutes
Frequency: Five times per week

Getting Started

Exercise programs are typically staged into pre-transplant, post-transplant, and home exercise programs. The pre-transplant and immediate post-transplant stages emphasize aerobic activities and maintain levels of physical function and strength.[1,5,6] Post-transplant and home exercise programs combine aerobic activities with resistance training to improve clients' physical function and quality of life and to decrease levels of fatigue.[1,7] During the first 100 post-transplant days, clients must avoid contact with the general public and are limited to hospital or home environments. Measures to prevent opportunistic infections are very important during this time. Post-transplant activities can be progressed to 70% to 80% of maximum heart rate for up to 30 minutes.[1] Resistance training programs are added to the aerobic activities in this stage and typically include lower- and upper-extremity movements with moderate intensity, using sets of 8 to 20 repetitions, beginning at 10 to 15 minutes and progressing to 30 minutes three times per week. Circuits that include leg and chest press exercises using pulley weight machines and free weight activities are commonly included in these programs.[1,7] Home-based exercise programs are important for improving clients' physical function and diminishing fatigue levels. Clients benefit from ongoing consultations to adjust their exercise program to ensure a complete recovery from their transplant procedure and to help prevent recurrence of their primary disease.

References

1. Wiskemann J, Huber G. Physical exercise as adjuvant therapy for patients undergoing hematopoietic stem cell transplantation. Bone Marrow Transplant 41(4):321-329, 2008.
2. Gillis TA, Donovan ES. Rehabilitation following bone marrow transplantation. Cancer 92(Suppl 4): 998-1007, 2001.
3. Bell LA, Epstein JB, Rose-Ped A, et al. Patient reports of complications of bone marrow transplantation. Support Care Cancer 8(1):33-39, 2000.
4. Jarden M, Baadsgaard MT, Hovgaard DJ, et al. A randomized trial on the effect of a multimodal intervention on physical capacity, functional performance and quality of life in adult patients undergoing allogeneic SCT. Bone Marrow Transplant 43(9):725-737, 2009.

5. Baumann FT, Kraut L, Schüle K, et al. A controlled randomized study examining the effects of exercise therapy on patients undergoing haematopoietic stem cell transplantation. Bone Marrow Transplant Jul 13, 2009.

6. Carlson LE, Smith D, Russell J, et al. Individualized exercise program for treatment of severe fatigue in patients after allogeneic hematopoietic stem-cell transplant: A pilot study. Bone Marrow Transplant 37(10):945-954, 2006.

7. Hayes SC, Davies PS, Parker TW, et al. Role of a mixed-type, moderate-intensity exercise programme after peripheral blood stem cell transplantation. Br J Sports Med 38(3):304-309, 2004.

CANCER, BONE TUMORS

Overview of Bone Tumors

Bony tumors are classified and named based on the type of tissue from which they originate: osteogenic, chondrogenic, fibrogenic, angiogenic, or myelogenic. The incidence for some bony tumors is associated with their location within a bone, the age of the client, and with certain types that are more prevalent in adolescents, who are undergoing rapid changes in their skeletal structures. Treatment of bone tumor is based on the location, size, and staging. Radiation and chemotherapies have been successfully used to treat many benign and metastatic tumors, whereas other tumors are best treated with surgical excision and limb salvage procedures.

Comorbidities to Consider

- Clients become deconditioned due to the disease process and treatment programs that produce persistent fatigue and decreased tolerance to physical activities.

Client Examination

Keys to Examination of Clients

- Determine the clients' physiologic status and preparedness for engaging in the physical activities by assessing the results of blood tests for platelet levels, hemoglobin, and white blood cell levels.
- As a general guideline, clients undergoing chemotherapy should not participate in aerobic activities when hemoglobin levels are <10 g/dL and platelet counts are <50,000/mm^3, but this may vary among medical centers. Clients need ongoing assessment for any abnormal responses to exercise.

Recommended Baseline Testing of Fitness Levels

- Use walking tests or a cycle ergometer to assess clients' tolerance for exercise.
- Clients' mobility and flexibility should be assessed before they begin exercise activities.[1] Clients who have undergone surgical procedures should be assessed for wound healing and potential for return to activities.
- Clients who have undergone amputation need to be assessed in preparation for prosthetic fitting or for wheelchair fitting. The Toronto Extremity Salvage Score or the Musculoskeletal Tumor Society Rating Scale can be used to provide a baseline for physical function, along with measures for pain and fatigue levels.[2-4]

Exercise Prescription

Type: Walking, cycle ergometry
Intensity: Low intensities, 40%–65% of maximum heart rate[5]
Duration: Start at 10–20 minutes, with short bouts
Frequency: Five times per week

Getting Started

Intensity should be assessed by heart rate and perceived exertion levels as fatigue may be a limiting factor. Emphasize full movements of the extremities during resistive exercises, using low resistance and high repetitions as these will be important for regaining range of motion and functional mobility.[5] Sitting and standing balance activities are important components for clients with amputated limbs in preparation for prosthetic or wheelchair fitting. Encourage clients to choose a variety of exercise and recreational activities to increase their levels of function and maintain a healthy lifestyle.

References

1. Carty CP, Dickinson IC, Watts MC, et al. Impairment and disability following limb salvage procedures for bone sarcoma. Knee 16(5):405-408, 2009.
2. Davis AM, Wright JG, Williams JI, et al. Development of a measure of physical function for patients with bone and soft tissue sarcoma. Quality Life Res 5(5):508-516, 1996.
3. Revised Musculoskeletal Tumor Society Rating Scale. http://faoj.files.wordpress.com/2009/03/fosstab1.pdf. Accessed November 23, 2009.
4. Davis AM, Punniyamoorthy S, Griffin AM, et al. Symptoms and their relationship to disability following treatment for lower extremity tumours. Sarcoma 3(2):73-77, 1999.
5. Adamsen L, Quist M, Andersen C, et al. Effect of a multimodal high-intensity exercise intervention in cancer patients undergoing chemotherapy: Randomised controlled trial. BMJ 339:b3410, 2009.

CANCER, BREAST

Overview of Breast Cancer

Breast cancer is the most common malignancy in women, with adenocarcinomas being the most common form of breast cancer. These carcinomas can affect breast ductal tissues and axillary lymph nodes, leading to malignancy. Treatment is based on the staging of the carcinoma and the client's hormonal sensitivity. Treatments usually include a combination of surgery, radiation and chemotherapies, and hormonal drugs. Clients become deconditioned due to the disease process and treatment programs that produce persistent fatigue and decreased tolerance to physical activities.[1,2]

Benefits of Exercise Programs for Clients With Breast Cancer

Improved cardiorespiratory fitness
Improved quality of life
Improved self-esteem

Improved physical functioning
Reduced fatigue
Improved rate of completion for chemotherapies

Comorbidities to Consider

- Damage to or removal of axillary lymph nodes during treatment increases the risk of clients developing an upper extremity lymphedema.[3]

Client Examination

Keys to Examination of Clients

- Determine clients' physiological status and preparedness for engaging in the physical activities by assessing results of blood tests for platelet levels, hemoglobin, and white blood cell levels.
- Clients undergoing chemotherapy may not be able to participate in aerobic activities when hemoglobin levels are <10 g/dL and platelet counts are <50,000/mm³.
- Clients who have undergone surgical excisions and other procedures may have limited mobility due to slowed wound healing and fibrotic scar formations.

Recommended Baseline Testing of Fitness Levels

- Use a walking or a cycle ergometer test to assess tolerance for exercise and to predict a Vo_2 maximum.
- Assess clients' mobility and flexibility before clients begin exercise activities. Clients who have undergone surgical removal of lymph nodes should have the upper extremities assessed for mobility; volumetric measures should be taken to assess for changes in edema levels.
- Upper- and lower-extremity strength can be assessed using hand weights, resistance tubing, or weight-lifting machines.
- Quality-of-life measures and fatigue levels can be assessed by the Functional Assessment of Cancer Therapy for breast cancer.[4,5]

Exercise Prescription

Type: Walking, cycling, aquatics, and resistance training[1,2,6-8]
Intensity: Start at 60% of Vo_2 maximum[2,6]
Duration: 15–20 minutes
Frequency: Three times per week

Getting Started

Exercise sessions can be used on days alternating with chemotherapy treatments. This allows clients to adapt to the exercise program while maintaining tolerance to adjuvant therapies for breast cancer. Yoga has been used to address persistent fatigue and emotional well-being.[9] Progressions of aerobic activities are recommended for up to 80% of Vo_2 maximum for 45 minutes, five times per week.[1,6] Resistance training is recommended for upper- and lower-extremity muscle groups at 60% to 70% of 1 repetition maximum for two sets of 8 to 12 repetitions three times per week. Clients who have completed their cancer treatments should be encouraged to maintain an aerobic exercise program to maintain fitness levels and help prevent a recurrence of breast cancer.[10] Clients can return to previous recreational activities when their overall fitness levels have returned to pre-treatment levels.

References

1. McNeely ML, Campbell KL, Rowe BH, et al. Effects of exercise on breast cancer patients and survivors: A systematic review and meta-analysis. CMAJ 175(1):34-41, 2006.
2. Courneya KS, Segal RJ, Mackey JR, et al. Effects of aerobic and resistance exercise in breast cancer patients receiving adjuvant chemotherapy: A multicenter randomized controlled trial. J Clin Oncol 25(28):4396-4404, October 1, 2007.
3. Meeske KA, Sullivan-Halley J, Smith AW, et al. Risk factors for arm lymphedema following breast cancer diagnosis in black women and white women. Breast Cancer Res Treat 113(2):383-391, 2009.
4. Functional assessment of cancer therapy. http://www.facit.org/about/welcome.aspx. Accessed February 5, 2010.
5. Bicego D, Brown K, Ruddick M, et al. Effects of exercise on quality of life in women living with breast cancer: A systematic review. Breast J 15(1):45-51, 2009.
6. Matthews CE, Wilcox S, Hanby CL, et al. Evaluation of a 12-week home-based walking intervention for breast cancer survivors. Support Care Cancer 15(2):203-211, 2007.
7. Portela ALM. Feasibility of an exercise progam for Puerto Rican women who are breast cancer survivors. Rehab Oncol 26(2):20-31, 2008.
8. Schmitz KH, Ahmed RL, Troxel A, et al. Weight lifting in women with breast–cancer-related lymphedema. NEJM 361(7):664-673, 2009.
9. Galantino ML. Potential benefits of walking and yoga on perceived levels of cognitive decline and persistent fatigue in women with breast cancer. Rehab Oncol 25(3):3-16, 2007.
10. Dorn J. Lifetime physical activity and breast cancer risk in pre- and postmenopausal women. Med Sci Sports Exerc 35(2):278-285, 2003.

CANCER, COLORECTAL

Overview of Colorectal Cancer

The most common types of colorectal cancers are adenocarcinomas and primary lymphomas. Adenocarcinomas begin in the mucosa of the colon and extend into the bowel wall. Progression of the disease affects the lymph nodes of the region, thus leading to metastases of the tumor. Surgical removal of the tumor by adjuvant chemotherapy is the most common treatment. Survival rates of clients diminish when the disease progresses to the lymph nodes. Physical inactivity has been identified as a significant risk factor for developing colorectal cancer.[1,2] Clients who develop this condition may already have limited endurance from a sedentary lifestyle.

Comorbidities to Consider

- Cardiovascular disease, hypertension, chronic obstructive pulmonary diseases, and diabetes mellitus are the most common comorbidities.[2]
- Clients recovering from colorectal cancer may have pain, fatigue, decreased immune function, and depression, which affects their physical activity level.[2]

Client Examination

Keys to Examination of Clients

- Clients with this condition will have undergone endoscopic examinations of the tumor and a blood test for the carcinoembryonic antigen.
- Assess clients' fatigue level and if clients suffer from other side effects related to their chemotherapy treatments.
- Discuss with clients the benefits of a regular exercise program as they may be resistant to changing their lifestyle to include exercise activities.[3]

Recommended Baseline Testing of Fitness Levels

- Use walking or cycle ergometer testing to assess for endurance levels and tolerance activities.
- Assess for postoperative pain and mobility limitations secondary to tumor removal.
- Use a behavioral change questionnaire to assess clients' readiness for participation in exercise activities.[4]

Exercise Prescription

Type: Walking, biking, recreational activities
Intensity: 65%–75% of predicted maximum heart.[5]
Duration: 20–30 minutes
Frequency: Five to six times per week

Getting Started

Moderate levels of physical activity have been found to reduce the risk significantly for recurrence of colorectal cancer and overall mortality.[6,7] Exercise parameters and reduced caloric intake promote weight loss and may greatly improve quality of life and survival rates.[2] Clients should be encouraged to maintain a regular exercise program to improve their quality of life and to prevent the recurrence of colorectal cancer.[6,7]

References

1. Slattery ML, Edwards S, Curtin K, et al. Physical activity and colorectal cancer. Am J Epidemiol 158(3):214-224, 2003.
2. Harriss DJ, Cable T, George K, et al. Physical activity before and after diagnosis of colorectal cancer. Sports Med 37(11):947-960, 2007.
3. Courneya KS, Friedenreich CM, Quinney HA, et al. A longitudinal study of exercise barriers in colorectal cancer survivors participating in a randomized controlled trial. Ann Behav Med 29(2):147-153, April 2005.
4. Marcus BH, Simkin, LR. The transtheoretical model: Applications to exercise behavior. Med Sci 1994. Sports Exerc 26:1400–1404.
5. Courneya KS, Friedenreich CM, Quinney HA, et al. A randomized trial of exercise and quality of life in colorectal cancer survivors. Eur J Cancer Care (Engl) 12(4):347-357, December 2003.
6. Meyerhardt JA, Heseltine D, Niedzweicki D, et al. Impact of physical activity on cancer recurrence and survival in patients with stage III colon cancer. J Clin Oncol 24(22):3535-3541, 2006.
7. Meyerhardt JA, Giovannucci EL, Holmes MD, et al. Physical activity and survival after colorectal cancer diagnosis. J Clin Oncol 22:3527-3534, 2006.

CANCER, HODGKIN LYMPHOMA

Overview of Hodgkin Lymphoma

This is a malignant lymphoma from the Reed-Sternberg cell found in the lymph nodes. Common sites of metastasis are the spleen, liver, and bone marrow. Clients are treated with combinations of radiation and chemotherapies. Although this type of lymphoma has a high cure rate, clients with a history of this condition may develop secondary cancers, long-term complications of cardiac diseases, and persistent fatigue.[1,2] Clients who are long-term survivors of this condition may have limited endurance due to the cardiotoxicity effects of radiation and chemotherapies on the myocardium.

Comorbidities to Consider

- Reduced activities and the effects of deconditioning limit clients' endurance.
- Clients with a history of smoking, hypercholesterolemia, and obesity have greater risk for heart disease.

Client Examination

Keys to Examination of Clients

- During acute stages, determine if activities need to be limited or restricted by assessing their white and red blood cell counts and levels of hemoglobin and hematocrit.
- Clients may undergo tests for heart and pulmonary function, including electrocardiogram, echocardiogram, stress testing, and spirometry.

Recommended Baseline Testing of Fitness Levels

- Assess for aerobic fitness with a walking or cycle ergometry test using small increments when increasing intensity.[3]
- Use strength and mobility tests to determine if clients will need to limit participation in exercise activities.[4,5]
- Assess fatigue level using the fatigue severity score.[6]

Exercise Prescription

Type: Treadmill walking or cycle ergometry in a hospital setting
Intensity: Start at 60% of maximum aerobic capacity[3,4]
Duration: 15–20 minutes
Frequency: Three times per week

Getting Started

Clients participating in a walking program can use low to moderate perceived exertion levels for 15 to 20 minutes with duration slowly progressed. Exercise parameters can be increased to 75% of maximum aerobic capacity for 45 minutes over a 2- to 3-month period.[3,4] Clients should be counseled to participate in regular exercise four to five sessions per week, with a goal of increasing to 150 minutes of exercise per week.[7] Long-term survivors of Hodgkin lymphomas may have heart and lung diseases and abnormal thyroid function that will limit their tolerance to exercise and limit their potential for improving physical function. Clients should be counseled to maintain a regular exercise program using different types of activities to maintain their adherence to and enjoyment of their program.

References

1. Aleman B, van Leeuwen F. Are we improving the long-term burden of Hodgkin's lymphoma patients with modern treatment? Hematol/Oncol Clin North Am 21(5):961-997, 2007.
2. Hjermstad MJ, Fosså SD, Oldervoll L, et al. Fatigue in long-term Hodgkin's disease survivors: A follow-up study. J Clin Oncol 23(27):6587-6595, 2005.
3. Fatigue Severity Score. http://www.mult-sclerosis.org/fatigueseverityscale.html. Accessed November 24, 2009.
4. Page E, Assouline D, Durand C, et al. Stage-related changes in functional capacity in Hodgkin's disease: Assessment by cardiopulmonary exercise testing before initiation of treatment. Ann Hematol 85(12): 857-861, 2006.
5. Courneya KS, Seller CM, Stevinson C, et al. Moderator effects in a randomized controlled trial of exercise training in lymphoma patients. Cancer Epidemiol Biomarkers Preview 18(10):2600-2607, 2009.
6. Courneya KS, Sellar CM, Stevinson C, et al. Randomized controlled trial of the effects of aerobic exercise on physical functioning and quality of life in lymphoma patients. J Clin Oncol 27(27):4605, 2009.
7. Vallance JK, Courneya KS, Jones LW, et al. Exercise preferences among a population-based sample of non-Hodgkin's lymphoma survivors. Eur J Cancer Care (Engl) 15(1):34-43, 2006.

CANCER, LEUKEMIA—ACUTE LYMPHOBLASTIC

Overview of Acute Lymphoblastic Leukemia

This condition is a malignant disease of the bone marrow and blood cells. The condition results in immature blast cells in the marrow and lymphoid organs, which limits development of normal blood cells. Clients may develop a variety of manifestations that include bleeding, bone pain, fatigue, and neurologic problems. The disease is found primarily in older adults with previous exposure to environmental hazards and infections. The treatment of this condition usually involves chemotherapy followed by bone marrow transplant, which requires extended hospitalization in an isolated environment.[1] Clients undergoing a bone marrow transplant will be confined in a hospital setting to prevent infections.

Environmental Risk Factors for Developing Acute Leukemia

Exposure to the chemical benzene
Infection of human leukocyte virus

Exposure to excessive levels of radiation
Long-term chemotherapies of alkylating agents

Comorbidities to Consider

- Neurologic problems of headaches, facial nerve palsy, blurred vision, and auditory abnormalities occur secondary to cerebral bleeding or leukemic infiltration of the brain.
- Clients develop limited endurance from anemia, loss of body mass, cancer-related fatigue, and depression.

Client Examination

Keys to Examination of Clients

- Exercise readiness can be determined by assessing the results of tests for blood counts, platelets, inflammatory markers, and hemoglobin levels. Low blood platelet levels ($<50,000/mm^3$) or low hemoglobin levels may preclude a client from participating in an exercise program.[2]
- Examine clients for arthralgias that may develop from leukemic infiltrates into the joint synovium.

Recommended Baseline Testing of Fitness Levels

- Use a cycle ergometer or treadmill walking test with a slow progression of exercise intensity to assess clients' cardiorespiratory endurance.[1,3]
- Clients' muscle strength and endurance can be tested by standard assessments or functional activities of squatting, stepping, or repetitive resisted movements.[1]

Exercise Prescription

Type: Walking, cycling, weight training
Intensity: Start with moderate levels of exercise followed by rest periods
Duration: 15–30 minutes
Frequency: Every other day or coordinated with chemotherapy treatments.

Getting Started

Use a treadmill or portable cycle ergometer and resistance exercises using hand weights, elastic bands, and other portable exercise equipment for clients confined to a hospital setting. Exercise programs have included a daily intermittent walking program starting at 70% of maximum heart rate for 3 minutes, followed by 3 minutes at half this intensity, for a total of 30 minutes.[3,4] Another program used cycle ergometry at 40% to 50% of heart rate reserve for up to 15 minutes, followed by 5 to 15 minutes of resistive exercise using hand weights and exercise balls and trunk-strengthening exercises.[1] This program was administered in a morning and afternoon session, followed by 36 hours of rest. Exercise was monitored by the client's perceived exertion level at <6 on the modified Borg scale CR10. Develop a home-walking and weight-training program for clients receiving outpatient chemotherapy. Remind clients undergoing treatment that fatigue levels will require extended rest periods between treatment and exercise sessions. Clients undergoing chemotherapy may experience periods of mood elevation and euphoria that may lead to excessive activities and overexertion.

Clients who have completed chemotherapy and/or bone marrow transplantations should be encouraged to maintain a regular exercise program to decrease the effects of their condition. Exercise programs during treatment have been found to diminish the effects of cancer-related fatigue and maintain quality-of-life measures.[1]

References

1. Battaglini CL, Hackney AC, Garcia R, et al. The effects of an exercise program in leukemia patients. Integrated Cancer Ther 8(2):130-138, 2009.
2. Elter T, Stipanov M, Heuser E, et al. Is physical exercise possible in patients with critical cytopenia undergoing intensive chemotherapy for acute leukaemia or aggressive lymphoma? Int J Hematol 90(2):199-204, 2009.
3. Dimeo F, Schwartz S, Fietz T, et al. Effects of endurance training on the physical performance of patients with hematological malignancies during chemotherapy. Support Care Cancer 11:623-628, 2003.
4. Chang PH, Lai YH, Shun SC, et al. Effects of a walking intervention on fatigue-related experiences of hospitalized acute myelogenous leukemia patients undergoing chemotherapy: A randomized controlled trial. J Pain Symptom Manage 35(5):524-534, 2008.

CANCER, LUNG

Overview of Lung Cancer

This condition includes many different types of tumors, with non–small cell lung cancer the most common type. Lung cancer is a leading cause of preventable death in the United States because smoking and environmental exposure are the primary risk factors. The risk of metastasis is high with these tumors due to the rich supply of lymphatic and blood vessels in the lungs. Treatment is usually a bout of radiation or chemotherapy, followed by surgical excision of the tumor. Clients become deconditioned due to the disease process and treatment programs that produce persistent fatigue and decreased tolerance to physical activities.

Comorbidities to Consider

- There is a high rate of complication with lung cancer that can affect the musculoskeletal structures of the trunk and upper extremities.
- Clients with a history of smoking or environmental exposures may have an underlying emphysema condition.

Client Examination

Keys to Examination of Clients

- Determine clients' physiologic status and preparedness for engaging in physical activities by assessing blood tests for platelet, hemoglobin, and white blood cell levels.
- Assessment of lung function helps determine clients' status for performing exercise testing and clients' capacity to improve aerobic capacity.
- Assess overall mobility of clients who have undergone surgical excisions; slowed wound healing and fibrotic scar formations can restrict movements.

Recommended Baseline Testing of Fitness Levels

- Use a cycle ergometer to measure peak Vo_2 and maximum heart rate.[1] A 6-minute walk test can assess exercise tolerance in clients undergoing chemotherapy for lung cancer.[2]
- Examine the breathing patterns and rib-cage expansion to determine if pulmonary rehabilitation interventions are needed.[3]
- Quality-of-life measures and fatigue levels can be assessed with the Functional Assessment of Cancer Therapy for lung cancer.[4]

Exercise Prescription

Type: Walking, stationary cycling
Intensity: Start at 60% of maximum heart rate[1,5,6]
Duration: 20–30 minutes
Frequency: 4 days per week, with a day of rest between each session

Getting Started

Alternate exercise days with chemotherapy days as fatigue will be a limiting factor for exercise activities. Progress the program over 4 weeks toward 70% of maximum Vo_2 or heart rate for 20 to 30 minutes 4 days per week. Exercise intensity is best assessed by a combination of heart rate measures and perceived exertion levels as fatigue levels may affect daily intensities of exercises. A low-intensity weight-training program can be added to an established aerobic fitness program. Clients undergoing chemotherapy will need to be managed for their level of fatigue and other side effects to maintain adherence to their exercise program.[7] Although treatment of this condition involves removal of or damage to lung parenchyma tissues, this may not significantly limit the client's exercise capacity.[1] Encourage clients who have recovered from treatment of lung cancer to maintain a regular program of exercise and recreational activities to improve their cardiopulmonary fitness and quality of life measures and to minimize the levels of fatigue.

References

1. Jones LW, Eves ND, Peterson BL, et al. Safety and feasibility of aerobic training on cardiopulmonary function and quality of life in postsurgical non-small cell lung cancer patients: A pilot study. Cancer 113(12):3430-3439, 2008.
2. Kasymjanova G, Correa JA, Kreisman H, et al. Prognostic value of the six-minute walk in advanced non-small cell lung cancer. J Thorac Oncol 4(5):602-607, 2009.
3. Nazarian J. Cardiopulmonary rehabilitation after treatment for lung cancer. Curr Treatment Options Oncol 5(1):75-82, 2004.
4. Functional Assessment of Cancer Therapy. http://www.facit.org/about/welcome.aspx. Accessed November 21, 2009.
5. Spruit MA, Janssen PP, Willemsen SC, et al. Exercise capacity before and after an 8-week multidisciplinary inpatient rehabilitation program in lung cancer patients: A pilot study. Lung Cancer 52(2):257-260, 2006.
6. Cesario A, Ferri L, Galetta D, et al. Postoperative respiratory rehabilitation after lung resection for non-small cell lung cancer. Lung Cancer. 57(2):175-180, 2007.
7. Ternel JS, Greer JA, Goldberg S, et al. A structured exercise program for patients with advanced non-small cell lung cancer. J Thorac Oncol 4(5):595-601, 2009.

CANCER, NON-HODGKIN LYMPHOMA

Overview of Non-Hodgkin Lymphoma

Non-Hodgkin lymphomas are a group of conditions that begin with the abnormal development of lymphocytes, resulting in solid tumors within the lymphatic system. Tumors usually arise in the lymph nodes, with malignant cells traveling via the lymphatic system to the thymus, spleen, and the gastrointestinal organs. Clients typically present with painless, enlarged lymph nodes, unexplained fever, and weight loss. Lymphomas may be aggressive or slow-growing. Treatment is with radiation and chemotherapies based on the staging of the disease, followed by a bone marrow transplant to reduce the size and activity of the lymphatic system tumors. Clients undergoing treatment for lymphomas typically have severe fatigue due to the disease process and the side effects of their treatment program.[1]

Comorbidities to Consider

• Clients who have undergone chemotherapy for aggressive types of lymphomas may develop impaired cardiac function.[2]

Client Examination

Keys to Examination of Clients

• Determine if physical activities need to be limited or restricted based on assessments of blood cell counts and hemoglobin and hematocrit levels. Clients undergoing treatment for lymphomas may be restricted from exercise activities if their white blood cell count is <5000/mm³, hemoglobin is <8 g/dL, or if platelets are <20,000/mm³.
• Clients receiving chemotherapy should have ongoing monitoring of their cardiac function during exercise testing.

Recommended Baseline Testing of Fitness Levels

• Endurance can be assessed using a 6-minute or 10-meter walk test depending on the client's environment and tolerance to activities.
• Examine clients for strength and mobility to determine if there will be activity limitations and if a type of exercise needs to be restricted.
• Assess fatigue levels using the Fatigue Severity Score.[3]

Exercise Prescription

Type: Walking, standing exercises[4]
Intensity: Start with low intensities
Duration: 10–30 minutes, depending on tolerance
Frequency: Three times per week

Getting Started

Clients should be encouraged to maintain some amount of standing and walking activities during treatment even though their fatigue level is persistent. After treatment, clients should be encouraged to participate in endurance activities to improve their cardiovascular health and quality of life.[5-7] Most clients prefer walking programs so that they can assess intensity using perceived exertion levels with the duration slowly progressed.[6] Clients should be counseled to participate in regular exercise in four to five sessions per week, with a goal of increasing to 150 minutes of moderate- to vigorous-level exercise per week.[4] Clients who have completed treatment should be encouraged to increase their physical activity level, as this will influence their health-related quality-of-life measures.[4]

References

1. Wang XS, Giralt SA, Mendoza TR, et al. Clinical factors associated with cancer-related fatigue in patients being treated for leukemia and non-Hodgkin's lymphoma. J Clin Oncol 20(5):1319-1328, 2002.
2. Elbl L, Vasova I, Tomaskova I, et al. Cardiac function and cardiopulmonary performance in patients after treatment for non-Hodgkin's lymphoma. Neoplasma 53(2):174-181, 2006.
3. Fatigue Severity Score. http://www.mult-sclerosis.org/fatigueseverityscale.html. Accessed November 24, 2009.
4. Bellizzi KM, Rowland JH, Arora NK, et al. Physical activity and quality of life in adult survivors of non-Hodgkin's lymphoma. J Clin Oncol 27(6):960-966, 2009.
5. Oldervoll LM, Loge JH, Kaasa S, et al. Physical activity in Hodgkin's lymphoma survivors with and without chronic fatigue compared with the general population: A cross-sectional study. BMC Cancer 7:210, 2007.
6. Vallance JK, Courneya KS, Jones LW, et al. Exercise preferences among a population-based sample of non-Hodgkin's lymphoma survivors. Eur J Cancer Care (Engl) 15(1):34-43, 2006.
7. Vallance JK, Courneya KS, Jones LW, et al. Differences in quality of life between non-Hodgkin's lymphoma survivors meeting and not meeting public health exercise guidelines. Psycho-oncology 14(11):979-991, 2005.

CANCER, OVARIAN

Overview of Ovarian Cancer

This is the second most common form of cancer in females, with most developing from an epithelial tumor. Most ovarian tumors are not detected until they are in an advanced stage and have metastasized as they produce only vague and nonspecific symptoms. Treatment usually involves a total hysterectomy and lymphadendectomy followed with chemotherapy. Clients who participate in the recommended levels of physical activities experience fewer complications related to the treatment of ovarian cancer.[1] Clients become deconditioned due to the disease process and treatment programs that produce persistent fatigue and decreased tolerance to physical activities. Many clients who have been diagnosed with ovarian cancer are older, have a history of high dietary fat intake, and lead a sedentary lifestyle.[2]

Comorbidities to Consider

- Clients may have urinary incontinence and significant weight loss and may develop a cerebellar degeneration that results in ataxia, nystagmus, and dysarthria.

Client Examination

Keys to Examination of Clients

- Determine clients' physiologic status and preparedness for engaging in physical activities by assessing the blood tests for platelet, hemoglobin, and white blood cell levels. Clients undergoing chemotherapy may be advised by their oncologist not to participate in aerobic activities when hemoglobin levels are <10 g/mL and platelet counts are <50,000/mm^3. Light exercise is permitted when platelet levels are between 20,000 and 30,000/mm^3.
- Examine overall mobility as clients who have undergone surgical excisions and other procedures may have limited mobility due to slowed wound healing and fibrotic scar formations.
- Discuss with clients their potential barriers to engaging in regular exercise activities.[2]

Common Barriers for Engaging in Exercise Activities

Lack of time	Lack of energy
Lack of motivation	Arthritis or joint problems
Comorbidities	Lack of equipment or facilities

Recommended Baseline Testing of Fitness Levels

- Use a walking test or a cycle ergometer test to assess clients' tolerance for exercise.
- Have clients perform tests for mobility and flexibility before beginning exercise activities.
- Quality-of-life measures and fatigue levels can be assessed with the Functional Assessment of Cancer Therapy for ovarian cancer.[3]

Exercise Prescription

Type: Walking, cycling, swimming[4]
Intensity: Start at 60% of predicted V_{O_2} maximum
Duration: 15–20 minutes
Frequency: Three times per week

Getting Started

Develop with the client an abdominal and pelvic floor strengthening routine that is started preoperatively and maintained postoperatively.[5] Exercise sessions can be used on days alternating with chemotherapy treatments. Resistance training can be combined with aerobic activities to improve muscle strength and improve quality of life. Progress aerobic activities to moderate intensities for 30 to 45 minutes three to five times per week.[1,6] Resistance training is recommended for upper- and lower-extremity muscle groups at 60% to 70% of one repetition maximum; for two sets of 8 to 12 repetitions two to three times per week.[6] Because obesity is a major risk factor for ovarian cancer, clients should maintain a regular exercise program with controlled diet for fat intake.[7]

References

1. Stevinson C, Steed H, Faught W, et al. Physical activity in ovarian cancer survivors: Associations with fatigue, sleep, and psychosocial functioning. Int J Gynecol Cancer 19(1):73-78, 2009.
2. Stevinson C, Tonkin K, Capstick V, et al. A population-based study of the determinants of physical activity in ovarian cancer survivors. J Phys Activity Health 6(3):339-346, 2009.
3. Functional Assessment of Cancer Therapy. http://www.facit.org/about/welcome.aspx. Accessed November 23, 2009.
4. Stevinson C, Capstick V, Schepansky A, et al. Physical activity preferences of ovarian cancer survivors. Psycho-oncology 18(4):422-428, 2009.
5. Watkins T, Maxeiner A. Musculoskeletal effects of ovarian cancer and treatment: A physical therapy perspective. Rehab Oncol 21(2):12, 2003.
6. Stevinson C, Faught W, Steed H, et al. Associations between physical activity and quality of life in ovarian cancer survivors. Gynecol Oncol 106(1):244-250, 2007.
7. Courneya KS, Karvinen KH, Campbell KL, et al. Associations among exercise, body weight, and quality of life in a population-based sample of endometrial cancer survivors. Gynecol Oncol 97(2):422-430, 2005.

CANCER, PROSTATE

Overview of Prostate Cancer

Prostate cancer is usually an adenocarcinoma that initially affects the outer prostate gland and then spreads inward with metastases in advanced stages. Risk factors include age greater than 50 years, African American race, and a family history of prostate cancer. Common treatments for prostate cancer include radical prostatectomy and radiation. Individuals in the advance stages of the disease may also receive androgen deprivation therapy to inhibit testosterone production. Individuals with prostate cancer may receive treatments that depress testosterone production, resulting in decreased physical function and fatigue.[1-3] Older men with early stages of the disease may not need treatment for this condition.[3] Those with advanced stages of this cancer or have undergone surgical procedures may experience back and pelvic pains with standing and walking activities, which may limit their daily activity levels.

Comorbidities to Consider

- Clients experiencing urinary incontinence with physical exertions may self-limit activities to avoid this problem.
- Symptoms of fatigue, weight loss, and dyspnea associated with physical activities have also been associated with symptoms for metastasis of the tumor.

Client Examination

Keys to Examination of Clients

- Ask your clients if they have had a recent test for their prostate antigen assay and prostatic acid phosphatase levels.
- Assess if your clients have symptoms of depression that may limit their preparedness to participate in exercise activities.[1,2] Screen clients in their 7th or 8th decade for cardiopulmonary conditions.

Recommended Baseline Testing of Fitness Levels

- Perform the 6-minute walk test to assess aerobic capacity and exercise tolerance.
- Measure upper and lower extremity strength levels to determine a baseline for resistive exercises.
- Measure fatigue using the Brief Fatigue Inventory or the Functional Assessment of Cancer Therapy for Fatigue.[4,5]

Exercise Prescription

Type: Walking, cycle ergometer, aquatic exercise[6,7]
Intensity: Start at 60%–70% of maximum heart rate
Duration: 20–30 minutes
Frequency: Three to four times per week.

Getting Started

Individuals experiencing urinary incontinence will benefit from pelvic floor exercises to improve the control of the external and internal sphincter muscles.[8] Clients with prostate cancer will have no restrictions for exercise directly related to this condition. Resistance training using a circuit of exercise for the upper and lower extremities has been beneficial for these clients.[7,9] Walking distance can be progressed to 45–60 minutes over a 12-week period. Resistance exercises for the upper and lower extremities can begin at 60%–70% of a one-rep maximum, with two sets of 8 to 12 repetitions.[6] Clients can return to previous recreational activities when their overall fitness levels have returned to pre-treatment levels.

References

1. Thorsen L, Courneya KS, Stevension C. et al. A systematic review of physical activity in prosate cancer survivors: Outcomes, prevalence, and determinants. Support Care Cancer 16:987-997, 2008.
2. Monga U, Garber SL, Thornby J, et al. Exercise prevents fatigue and improves quality of life in prostate cancer patients undergoing radiotherapy. Arch Phys Med Rehabil 88:1416-1422, 2007.
3. Clay CA, Perera S, Wagner JM, et al. Physical function in men with prostate cancer on androgen deprivation therapy. Phys Ther 87(10):1325-1333, 2007.
4. Mendoza TR, Wang XS, Cleeland CS, et al. The rapid assessment of fatigue severity in cancer patients: Use of the Brief Fatigue Inventory. Cancer 85:1186-1196, 1999.
5. Webster K, Cella D, Yost K. The functional assessment of chronic illness therapy measurement system: Properties, applications, and interpretation. Health Qual Life Outcomes 79:1, 2003.
6. Segal RJ, Reid RD, Courneya KS, et al. Randomized controlled trial of resistance or aerobic exercise in men receiving radiation therapy for prostate cancer. J Clin Oncol 27:344-351, 2009.
7. Windsor PM, Nicol KF, Potter J. A randomized, controlled trial of aerobic exercise for treatment-related fatigue in men receiving radical external beam radiotherapy for localized prostate carcinoma. Cancer 101:550-557, 2004.
8. MacDonald R, Fink HA, Huckaby C, et al. Pelvic floor muscle training to improve urinary incontinence after radical prostatectomy: A systematic review of effectiveness. BJU Int 100:76-81, 2007.
9. Segal RJ, Reid RD, Courneya KS, et al. Resistance exercise in men receiving androgen deprivation therapy for prostate cancer. J Clin Oncol 21:1653-1659, 2003.

CHRONIC FATIGUE SYNDROME

Overview of Chronic Fatigue Syndrome

This condition is an unexplained, persistent fatigue that is not a result of exertion and that lasts for 6 months or longer. Clients typically have unexplained fatigue along with symptoms of diffuse pain with impaired memory or concentration. This condition can result from numerous biologic, behavioral, and psychological factors. The leading cause is hypothesized to be the presence of a chronic infection that induces changes to the immunologic and neuroendocrine functions and autonomic nervous system regulation.[1]

Unexplained fatigue for fewer than 6 months is called prolonged fatigue. Clients with this condition experience abnormal responses to exercise activities that result in debilitating fatigue that is not reversed with rest or sleep. Their abnormal endocrinologic and immunologic responses produce fatigue that leads to significant deficits in endurance and cardiopulmonary functions. Prolonged inactivity in poorly supported seated positions can lead to altered trunk postures and abnormal breathing patterns. Clients will learn to limit their activity levels to avoid fatigue symptoms and develop avoidance behaviors that result in reluctance to participate in exercise.[2]

Comorbidities to Consider

• Clients may also have a variety of physical symptoms with this condition.[1]

Concurrent Symptoms That May Occur With Chronic Fatigue Syndrome

Sore throat	Memory loss
Tender lymph nodes	Muscle pain
Arthralgias	Headaches
Unrefreshing sleep	Postexertional malaise

Client Examination

Keys to Examination of Clients

• Discuss with your clients what type of testing has been performed to rule out other conditions.
• Monitor the results of tests for blood counts and chemistry for signs of infection.

Recommended Baseline Testing of Fitness Levels

• Perform tests of vital signs and perceived exertion ratings before and after testing sessions.
• Examine clients in sitting and standing positions for breathing patterns, dyspnea, and hypotension.
• Have clients assess their fatigue level on a 1–10 scale before exercise and at intervals after exercise.[1]

Exercise Prescription

Type: Standing activities, walking, postural exercises
Intensity: Begin with very low levels of activities
Duration: Start with intermittent periods of 2–3 minutes
Frequency: Daily as tolerated

Getting Started

The combination of graded submaximal aerobic exercise and cognitive behavior therapy is the best method for improving activity levels and lessening fatigue symptoms.[3-5] Begin exercise sessions with stretching activities and exercises for improving posture and breathing patterns. Exercise sessions may need to be started with only minimal durations of exercise along with encouragement for the client to increase daily activities that involve standing and walking activities. Closely monitor vital signs and perceived exertion levels, but do not use perceived exertion or fatigue levels during exercise to grade or progress exercise as these clients have become unable to use internal cues to grade their exercise capacity, which could result in overexertion.[5] Clients with this condition will need close monitoring so that exercise intensity and duration are appropriately prescribed and progressed. Clients with chronic fatigue syndrome will need to learn self-management methods to determine how much activities are appropriate for improving their activity levels and diminishing fatigue. Graded progressions in exercise will need to be made through ongoing interaction with the client.

References

1. Center for Disease Control. Chronic fatigue syndrome. http://www.cdc.gov/cfs/cfsdefinitionHCP.htm Accessed November 24, 2009.
2. Wallman KE, Morton AR, Goodman C, et al. Physiological responses during a submaximal cycle test in chronic fatigue syndrome. Med Sci Sports Exerc 36(10):1682-1688, 2004.
3. Edmonds M, McGuire H, Price J. Exercise therapy for chronic fatigue syndrome. Cochrane Database Syst Rev 3:CD003200, 2004.
4. Price JR, Mitchell E, Tidy E, et al. Cognitive behavior therapy for chronic fatigue syndrome in adults. Cochrane Database Syst Rev 3:CD001027, 2008.
5. Nijs J, Paul L, Wallman K. Chronic fatigue syndrome: An approach combining self-management with graded exercise to avoid exacerbations. J Rehabil Med 40(4):241-247, 2008.

CHRONIC OBSTRUCTIVE PULMONARY DISEASE (COPD)

Overview of Chronic Obstructive Pulmonary Disease

This condition refers to disorders that affect movement of air into and out of the lungs, with emphysema and chronic bronchitis being the most common disorders. Clients develop limitations of the pulmonary and cardiovascular systems, skeletal muscle dysfunctions, nutritional impairments, and increasing levels of anxiety or fear. Treatment combines medical therapies, medications, oxygen therapy, and rehabilitation programs to control the client's symptoms and to limit progression of the disease. Clients experience dyspnea, leg fatigue, and discomfort with physical exertions, which result in a decrease in activities as the disease progresses. Dyspnea is created by the client's inability to expire air from the lungs.

Comorbidities to Consider

- Clients in advanced stages have signs of deconditioning, respiratory muscle shortening, and lower extremity muscle weakness.[1]

Client Examination

Keys to Examination of Clients

- Assess the results of pulmonary function testing to determine levels of airflow limitations; use the reduction of forced expiratory volume as a key measurement for monitoring changes in the disease process.
- Measure clients' level of dyspnea by using a 0–5 scale.[2]
- Before starting exercise testing, assess clients' trunk and rib cage mobility and tolerance for sitting positions.
- Before starting exercise testing, assess the use of pursed-lip breathing and medications.

Recommended Baseline Testing of Fitness Levels

- A cycle ergometry endurance test is the most common method for assessing cardiopulmonary response to exercises. A 6-minute walk test and treadmill walking have also been used to assess endurance.
- Strength testing, especially for the quadriceps muscle group, can be assessed with one repetition maximum test using a hand or isokinetic dynamometer.[3]

Exercise Prescription

Type: Cycle ergometer, treadmill walking
Intensity: Start at low intensities of 50%–60% of work maximums
Duration: Start at 10–20 minutes
Frequency: Three times per week

Getting Started

Clients with uncontrolled dyspnea will be restricted from participating in an exercise program. Clients with chronically high levels of CO_2 (hypercapnia) may respond poorly to exercise activities. Clients with severe congestive heart failure and pulmonary hypertension are not permitted to engage in exercise programs. If a client develops excessive anxiety or mental instability with increasing levels of dyspnea, restrict the client from participating in the exercise program until efforts to control these problems are successful.[1] Progress exercise sessions to 30 minutes of continuous exercise.[3] Interval training has been used to improve tolerance to physical activities by alternating short bouts of 30–60 seconds of high-intensity cycling, followed by rest of similar length.[1] Strength training using low-intensity workloads have used two to four sets of 20 repetitions to improve muscle strength and tolerance to physical activities.[2,4] Breathing exercises using hyperventilation while re-breathing CO_2 have been used to mimic the load on respiratory muscles during exercise activities.[5] Supplemental oxygen therapy is typically not used during these exercise programs but may benefit clients who become excessively hypoxic as they begin their exercise program.[6] Clients should learn how to maintain their exercise program independently, as the benefits of a formal exercise program will be lost if exercise activities are stopped.[1]

References

1. Rochester CL. Exercise training in chronic obstructive pulmonary disease. J Rehabil Res Dev 40(5 Suppl 2):59-80, 2003.
2. http://www.copd-international.com/Library/stages.htm. Accessed November 22, 2009.
3. Puhan MA, Schunemann HJ, Frey M, et al. How should COPD patients exercise during respiratory rehabilitation? Comparison of exercise modalities and intensities to treat skeletal muscle dysfunction. Thorax 60(5):367-375, 2005.
4. Ries AL. Pulmonary rehabilitation: Summary of an evidence-based guideline. Respir Care 53(9):1203-1207, 2008.
5. Mador MJ, Deniz O, Aggarwal A, et al. Effect of respiratory muscle endurance training in patients with COPD undergoing pulmonary rehabilitation. Chest 128(3):1216-1224, 2005.
6. Nonoyama ML, Brooks D, Lacasse Y, et al. Oxygen therapy during exercise training in chronic obstructive pulmonary disease. Cochrane Database Syst Rev 2:CD005372, 2007.

CHRONIC RENAL FAILURE

Overview of Chronic Renal Failure

Chronic renal failure is due to the loss of the kidney's nephrons, which results in diminished filtration and endocrine functions. Chronic renal failure is assessed by measures of glomerlular filtration rates. Hypertension and diabetes mellitus are the two most common causes of renal failure, with renal failure significantly affecting other systems of the body. Hereditary defects of the kidneys, urinary tract infections, age, and excessive use of analgesics are risk factors for this condition. Individuals with less than 10% of kidney function are in end-stage renal disease and require dialysis. Individuals with renal failure may have anemia, diminished oxygen transport, and decreased ability to maintain blood volumes, which result in fatigue and dyspnea with physical exertion.

Comorbidities to Consider

• Renal failure is associated with hypertension, heart disease, and diabetes mellitus.

Client Examination

Keys to Examination of Clients

• Determine blood urea nitrogen and serum creatinine levels, but changes in these levels do not usually restrict participation in exercise activities.
• Individuals with end-stage renal disease may have low levels of function, which limit the types and amount of baseline testing.

Recommended Baseline Testing of Fitness Levels

• Self-paced walking, treadmill walking, and cycle ergometer tests are the preferred methods.[1-3]
• Individuals with chronic renal failure usually have hypertension and heart disease, which are significant precautions for exercise programs.

Exercise Prescription

Type: Walking, treadmill walking, cycle ergometry
Intensity: Low to moderate levels
Duration: Start at 10–15 minutes
Frequency: Three times per week

during

Getting Started

Walking programs and cycle ergometers are the best modes of exercise for clients with renal failure. Those receiving dialysis may choose to exercise on dialysis or on non-dialysis days. Clients taking dialysis can perform exercise using a treadmill, cycle ergometer, or bed/chair exercises. Greater improvements in physical and cardiopulmonary function have been found for those who exercise on non-dialysis days, but exercise during dialysis can be an effective and more efficient means for ensuring adherence to the exercise program.[4,5]

Recommended levels of aerobic activities are within 60% to 70% of maximum heart rate, with frequent assessment of blood pressure and perceived exertion.[5] Exercise programs should consist of a long warm-up followed by a consistent level of effort during aerobic and strengthening activities. A cool-down period is also important to allow for return of fluid distribution and blood pressure. Clients should learn to assess their exercise intensity level primarily by their rate of perceived exertion and not by heart rate.[6] Lightheadedness, dizziness, pain, and dyspnea are indicators that exercise needs to be stopped and the client reassessed.[3] Progressions of exercise should be gradual, with frequent assessments to determine the appropriate level. Long-term adoption of exercise behaviors are needed by individuals with renal failure, as these activities are important for maintaining functional capacities and quality of life.[7]

References

1. Painter P. Determinants of exercise capacity in CKD patients treated with hemodialysis. Adv Chronic Kidney Dis 16(6):437-448, 2009.
2. Johansen KL. Exercise and dialysis. Hemodial Int 12:290-300, 2008.
3. Evans N, Forsyth E. End-stage renal disease in people with type 2 diabetes: Systemic manifestations and exercise implications. Phys Ther 84:454-463, 2004.
4. Kouidi E, Grekas D, Deligiannis A, et al. Outcomes of long-term exercise training in dialysis patients: Comparison of two training programs. Clin Nephrol. 61(Suppl 1):S31-38, 2004.
5. Konstantinidou E, Koukouvou G, Kouidi E, et al. Exercise training in patients with end-stage renal disease on hemodialysis: Comparison of three rehabilitation programs. J Rehabil Med 34(1):40-45, 2002.
6. Fuhrmann I, Krause R. Principles of exercising in patients with chronic kidney disease, on dialysis and for kidney transplant recipients. Clin Nephrol. 61(Suppl 1):S14-25, 2004.
7. Levendoğlu F, Altintepe L, Okudan N, et al. A twelve week exercise program improves the psychological status, quality of life and work capacity in hemodialysis patients. J Nephrol 17(6):826-832, 2004.

CHRONIC VENOUS INSUFFICIENCY

Overview of Chronic Venous Insufficiency

This condition is a decreased venous return due to venous stasis and increased venous pressures from damage to vein valves. Clients with this condition typically have a history of chronic venous inflammation and vein thrombosis. The condition results in venous hypertension due to excessive fluids in the veins, leading to fluids and whole blood cells migrating into the interstitial spaces. Clients exhibit edema in the legs and ankles, degenerative changes in the skin, and possibly ulcerations. Clients may have open wounds in the distal leg and need proper wound care and ongoing assessment of the legs, ankles, and feet for signs of increasing edema and skin breakdown. Clients experience fatigue as well as aching and heaviness in the legs with walking activities due to inadequate return of blood flow to heart and lungs. Clients typically adopt slower walking velocities that may lead to diminished plantarflexor muscle endurance and decreased plantar flexor muscle lengths.[1] Diminished walking activities will lead to decreased daily activities and limited endurance.

Comorbidities to Consider

- Clients may also have heart disease, diabetes mellitus, intermittent claudication, or a history of leg skin burns and grafting.

Client Examination

Keys to Examination of Clients

- Clients can be assessed with Doppler arterial blood flow studies and brachial and ankle blood pressures.
- Air plethysmography assesses the venous flow from the legs and the amount of venous reflux.
- Clients with a history of heart disease need ongoing monitoring of vital signs and for physical signs of congestive heart failure.

Recommended Baseline Testing of Fitness Levels

- Client's exercise tolerance is best assessed with the 6-minute walk test for endurance or the 10-meter walk velocity test.
- Assess the severity of the client's venous insufficiency with the venous severity score.[2]
- Use the standing heel raise test or a dynamometer to assess the strength of the ankle plantar flexor muscles.
- Motion at the ankle joint and gastrocnemius-soleus muscle length and fitness should be assessed before starting strength testing activities.
- Inspect the lower extremity skin, and assess for pain and edema to determine the client's present condition and to determine if these signs have changed during treatment.

Exercise Prescription

Type: Walking, standing exercises
Intensity: Moderate pace
Duration: 5–10-minute periods
Frequency: Daily

Getting Started

A supervised program of calf muscle stretching, lower extremity strengthening activities, and walking has been used to increase activity levels and to improve venous return from the legs.[3,4] A calf or plantar flexor muscle strengthening program using standing heel raising exercises has been used to improve muscle strength and leg venous return levels.[5] Heel raising exercises can begin with clients performing half the repetitions of their maximum number for three sets, with 3 to 5 minutes of rest between sets. Walking uphill has been used to promote plantar flexor strength and improve walking distances. These exercise sessions can be performed every other day.[6] Clients should be encouraged to exercise with compression stockings to improve the venous flow through the legs, promote oxygenation of deeper tissues, and to minimize the amount of reflux after their exercise session.[4,7] Activities that require prolonged standing and sitting should be avoided, and any activity that requires vigorous or ballistic movement through the lower extremities will be contraindicated.[8] Clients can be progressed from supervised programs to independent programs, with periodic assessment of fitness and for tests of venous return. Clients should be encouraged to maintain the strength and endurance of ankle plantar flexors as they serve as a dynamic pump for return of blood flow during standing and walking activities.

References

1. van Unden C. Gait and calf muscle endurance in patients with chronic venous insufficiency. Clin Rehab 19(3):339-445, 2005.
2. Vasquez MA, Munschauer CE. Venous clinical severity score and quality-of-life assessment tools: Application to vein practice. Phlebology 23(6):259-275, 2008.
3. Padberg FT, Johnston MV, Sisto SA. Structured exercise improves calf muscle pump function in chronic venous insufficiency: A randomized trial. Vascular 39(1):79-87, 2004.
4. Zajkowski PJ, Draper T, Bloom J, et al. Exercise with compression stockings improves reflux in patients with mild chronic venous insufficiency. Phlebology 21(2):100-104, 2006.
5. Kan YM, Delis KT. Hemodynamic effects of supervised calf muscle exercise in patients with venous leg ulceration: A prospective controlled study. Arch Surg 136(12):1364-1369, 2001.
6. Yang YK, Vandongen YK, Stacey MC. Effect of exercise on calf muscle pump function in patients with chronic venous disease. Br J Surg 86(3):338-341, 1999.
7. Agu O, Baker D, Seifalian AM. Effect of graduated compression stockings on limb oxygenation and venous function during exercise in patients with venous insufficiency. Vascular 12(1):69-76, 2004.
8. Rathbun SW, Kirkpatrick AC. Treatment of chronic venous insufficiency. Curr Cardiovascular Med 9: 115-126, 2007.

CIRRHOSIS

Overview of Cirrhosis

This condition is the end-stage disease of the liver resulting from a variety of diseases, most commonly hepatitis C and alcohol abuse. Cirrhosis of the liver tissue is from inflammation, fibrotic scarring, and obstruction of biliary channels. These changes lead to jaundice, portal hypertension, and decreased clearing of waste from the blood. Clients experience more fatigue, malnutrition, and muscle cramping as the disease progresses.[1] Fatigue is related to significant reduction in muscle mass and strength and increased presence of ammonia in the circulating plasma.[2,3] At end-stage, the client develops ascites of the abdomen and edema in the lower extremities, which may significantly reduce the client's daily activities.

Comorbidities to Consider

- Diminished aerobic capacity is related to myocardial thickening, limited pulmonary function, and inability to increase cardiac output during activities.[4,5]
- Clients often develop diabetes and display greatly reduced cardiovascular and skeletal muscle functions.[2,4]

Client Examination

Keys to Examination of Client

- Discuss clients' problems with mobility and fatigue.
- Ask clients if they have symptoms of abdominal pain, muscle cramping, nausea, and nutritional intake before recommending an exercise program.

Recommended Baseline Testing of Fitness Levels

- Use a 6-minute walk test or a 10-meter velocity test as a baseline for endurance.
- Assessments of mobility, muscle strength, and fatigue levels establish a baseline for physical activities.

Exercise Prescription

Type: Walking, treadmill walking, cycle ergometry
Intensity: Low to moderate intensities[1,6]
Duration: 5–10-minute bouts with rest periods
Frequency: Three to four times per week

Getting Started

Clients with well-compensated liver disease should be encouraged to participate in mild to moderate exercise programs.[6,7] Ongoing evaluation of the condition is needed to adjust the exercise program to limit any complications secondary. Clients can be advised to exercise for short periods with rest breaks using their perceived exertion levels to adjust the daily intensity level. The client should be assessed for abdominal swelling and edema in the lower extremities during and after exercise. Abdominal pain, vomiting of blood, and increased distention of abdominal veins are possible signs of portal hypertension. Clients who have developed ascites that is not controlled with diuretics will be restricted from exercise activities. Clients with well-compensated liver disease should be encouraged to increase the duration and frequency of their exercise activities. Long-term adaption of exercise activities may serve to improve quality of life measures and the client's sense of well-being.[7,8]

References

1. Kato S, Onishi S, Yamazaki H. Skeletal muscle in liver disease. In Skeletal Muscle: Pathology, Diagnosis and Management, ed. Preedy and Peters. Cambridge University Press, 2002.
2. Andersen H, Borre M, Jakobsen J, et al. Decreased muscle strength in patients with alcoholic liver cirrhosis in relation to nutritional status, alcohol abstinence, liver function, and neuropathy. Hepatology 27(5):1200-1206, 1998.
3. Dietrich R, Bachmann C, Lauterburg BH. Exercise-induced hyperammonemia in patients with compensated chronic liver disease. Scand J Gastroenterol 25(4):329-334, 1990.
4. Wong F, Girgrah N, Graba J, et al. The cardiac response to exercise in cirrhosis. Gut 49(2):268-275, 2001
5. Epstein SK, Zilberberg MD, Jacoby C, et al. Response to symptom-limited exercise in patients with the hepatopulmonary syndrome. Chest 114(3):736-741, 1998.
6. Saló J, Guevara M, Fernández-Esparrach G, et al. Impairment of renal function during moderate physical exercise in cirrhotic patients with ascites: Relationship with the activity of neurohormonal systems. Hepatology 25(6):1338-1342, 1997.
7. Cortez-Pinto H, Machado M. Impact of body weight, diet and lifestyle on nonalcoholic fatty liver disease. Expert Rev Gastroenterol Hepatol 2(2):217-231, 2008.
8. Bellentani S, Dalle Grave R, et al. Behavior therapy for nonalcoholic fatty liver disease: The need for a multidisciplinary approach. Hepatology 47(2):746-754, 2008.

CONGESTIVE HEART FAILURE

Overview of Heart Failure

This condition is due to the heart being unable to supply enough blood to the body's tissues. The lungs are significantly affected as a backup of blood in the pulmonary veins leads to pulmonary hypertension. This condition also affects the function of numerous organs and tissues. Heart failure is usually the consequence of ischemic and hypertensive heart disease. There are four types of heart failure, based on the cause and location of myocardium damage. The Functional Classification of Heart Failure, based on the client's tolerance to physical activities, is used to help determine the progression of the disease.[1,2] Treatment is focused on the primary cause of the condition, using diet, medication, and exercise to manage it. Some clients will have undergone heart valve replacement, coronary artery bypass grafting, or heart reduction surgery. Clients experience significant dyspnea and fatigue with physical activities due to the heart's inability to adequately supply blood to extremities, which in turn leads to atrophy of extremity muscles.[1]

Functional Classification of Heart Failure

Class I: Mild—Ordinary physical activity does not result in fatigue, palpitation, or dyspnea

Class II: Mild—Ordinary physical activity results in fatigue, palpitation, or dyspnea

Class III: Moderate—Comfortable at rest, but less than ordinary activity causes fatigue, palpitation, or dyspnea

Class IV: Severe—Unable to carry out any physical activity without discomfort

Comorbidities to Consider

- Clients may experience significant weight gain and peripheral edema that will affect their mobility.

Client Examination

Keys to Examination of Clients

- Clients have undergone numerous tests for heart and lung function.
- Perform frequent assessments of vital signs and heart and lung sounds to determine clients' tolerance to exercise activities.
- Discuss with clients their barriers and potential barriers to beginning and maintaining a regular exercise program.[3]

Recommended Baseline Testing of Fitness Levels

- Treadmill walking and the 6-minute walk test are common methods for measuring exercise tolerance and assessing cardiopulmonary function.
- Muscle strength and functional mobility are important to assess for clients with moderate to severe (class III and IV) heart failure.[1,2]
- Measure clients' dyspnea and fatigue levels before and during exercise sessions.

Exercise Prescription

Type: Walking, treadmill walking, cycle ergometry[3]
Intensity: Start at 50% of Vo_2 maximum or heart rate reserve[3,4]
Duration: Start with short bouts with rest periods
Frequency: Three to four times per week.

Getting Started

Clients with mild to moderate heart failure (class II and III) can begin an endurance exercise program at 50% of maximum Vo_2 or their heart rate reserve.[3,4] Short bouts of 10 minutes of exercise, followed by a rest period, are appropriate for beginning the exercise program. Exercise intensities can be advanced to up to 70% of maximum Vo_2. Progression of intensity is based on the client's physiologic tolerance to the activity. The effects of resistive exercise for improving heart function has been controversial, but resistive exercises can be combined with endurance training with no detrimental effects on heart or lung function.[5,6] Resistive exercise can begin at 50% of a one-repetition maximum, with one set of 10 to 15 repetitions. Progression of resistive exercise is with small incremental increases while maintaining full movements.[3,7]

Clients with uncontrolled hypertension and cardiac arrhythmias will be precluded from starting an exercise program, but even clients with severe heart failure can benefit from an exercise prescription. Exercise programs need to be progressed to an independent program for each client. Clients need to choose their own preference of exercise and recreational activities to maintain their cardiorespiratory fitness and quality of life.[4] Clients must be taught to monitor key symptoms (e.g., breathlessness, fatigue, and swelling) using a scale from 1 to 5 and to report new or worsening symptoms. Waiting too long to seek help can lead to cessation of an active exercise program along with significant morbidity and even death.

References

1. Cahalin LP. Heart failure. Phys Ther 76(5):516-533, 1996.
2. Russell SD, Saval MA, Robbins JL, et al. New York Heart Association functional class predicts exercise parameters in the current era. Am Heart J. 158(4 Suppl):S24-30, 2009.
3. Mandic S, Tymchak W, Kim D, et al. Effects of aerobic or aerobic and resistance training on cardiorespiratory and skeletal muscle function in heart failure: A randomized controlled pilot trial. Clin Rehabil 23(3):207-216, 2009.
4. Riegel B, Moser DK, Anker SD, et al. State of the science: Promoting self-care in persons with heart failure: A scientific statement from the American Heart Association. Circulation 120(12):1141-1163, 2009.
5. Bartlo P. Evidence-based application of aerobic and resistance training in patients with congestive heart failure. J Cardiopulmonary Rehabil Prev 27(6):368-375, 2007.
6. Spruit MA, Eterman RM, Hellwig VA, et al. Effects of moderate-to-high intensity resistance training in patients with chronic heart failure. Heart 95(17):1399-1408, 2009.
7. Beckers PJ, Denollet J, Possemiers NM, et al. Combined endurance-resistance training vs. endurance training in patients with chronic heart failure: A prospective randomized study. Eur Heart J 29(15):1858-1866, 2008.

CORONARY ARTERY DISEASE (CAD)

Overview of CAD

CAD develops as a result of progressive narrowing of coronary arteries, which leads to ischemia of the heart muscle. Atherosclerosis is the most common cause for narrowing of the coronary arteries, with numerous other causes of narrowing and obstructions. A number of risk factors have been identified, including physical inactivity, obesity, hypertension, and hypercholesterolemia. Narrowing of the coronary arteries can be treated with a wide range of medications and through angioplasty procedures. Exercise programs have been shown to significantly improve the total mortality of clients with CAD.[1] Clients develop impaired endurance due to the heart's inability to maintain blood flow to the myocardium, which limits the heart's ability to increase blood flow to the lungs and extremities.[2]

Benefits of Exercise Programs for Coronary Arteries

Improved endothelial function	Improved myocardial oxygen demand
Improved autonomic tone	Development of coronary collateral arteries
Decreased inflammatory markers	Decreased clotting factors

Comorbidities to Consider

- Clients may have symptoms of chest pain, palpitations, dyspnea, and fatigue related to this condition.

Client Examination

Keys to Examination of Clients

- Clients may have undergone stress testing along with imaging of their cardiac circulation and heart function.
- Clients need ongoing assessments of their blood pressure, heart rhythms, and heart rate.

Recommended Baseline Testing of Fitness Levels

- Aerobic capacity can be assessed with graded exercise testing, walking, and cycling tests.
- Estimate resistance training levels using one repetition or 10-repetition maximum testing.[2]

Exercise Prescription

Type: Walking, treadmill walking, cycle ergometry[3,4]
Intensity: 60%–80% of maximum heart rate[3,5]
Duration: 30 minutes
Frequency: Five times per week

Getting Started

Aerobic activities can be started with two 20-minute bouts of exercise, with a 10-minute rest period. Heart rate is not recommended as the sole determinant for measuring the intensity of exercises, as many clients use a beta-blocker drug that diminishes the heart rate response to activities and limits blood pressure and myocardial contractility. A client's rate of perceived exertion at a level of 12 to 16 can be used in conjunction with heart rate measurements. Resistance training with the upper and lower extremities has been used in combination with aerobic exercises.[6] A circuit of resistance training of 8 to 10 upper and lower exercises can be prescribed using 2 to 3 sets of 15 repetitions at 60% of a one-repetition maximum, using 30 to 60-second rest periods between sets.[6,7] Resistive training that emphasizes eccentric muscle contractions has been proposed as a method that produces muscle strength changes with less demand on cardiovascular function.[8] Aquatic exercise has also been used for improving the exercise tolerance in CAD clients. Aquatic exercise can be performed 50% to 70% of maximal heart rate for 30 to 40 minutes, with a 10-minute warm-up and cool down period.[7]

Clients with a history of chest pain during physical activities may be reluctant to begin an exercise program. The risk for sudden death and myocardial infarction is greatest for sedentary adults participating in unaccustomed, vigorous physical activities.[3] Clients may need to use a nitrate vasodilator in the event of chest pain or angina. Calcium channel blockers dilate coronary arteries to lower blood pressure and suppress arrhythmias. Clients need to be counseled to maintain a long-term exercise program to maintain fitness and to attain improvements in endothelial lining of the coronary arteries and improve microcirculation of the myocardium.[4]

References

1. Taylor RS, Brown A, Ebarahim S, et al. Exercise-based rehabilitation for patients with coronary heart disease: Systematic review and meta-analysis of randomized controlled trials. Am J Med 116(10):682-692, 2004.
2. Fletcher GF, Balady GJ, Amsterdam EA, et al. Exercise standards for testing and training: A statement for healthcare professionals from the American Heart Association. Circulation 104(14):1694-1740, 2001.
3. Thompson PD, Buchner D, Pina I, et al. Exercise and physical activity in the prevention and treatment of atherosclerotic cardiovascular disease. Circulation 107:3109-3116, 2003.
4. Gielen S, Schuler G, Hambrecht R. Exercise training in coronary artery disease and coronary vasomotion. Circulation Jan 2:103(1):E1-6l, 2001.
5. Hansen D, Dendale P, Berger J, et al. Importance of exercise training session duration in the rehabilitation of coronary artery disease patients. Eur J Cardiovasc Prev Rehabil 15(4):453-459, 2008.
6. Marzolini S, Oh PI, Thomas SG, et al. Aerobic and resistance training in coronary disease: Single versus multiple sets. Med Sci Sports Exerc 40(9):1557-1564, 2008.
7. Volaklis KA, Spassis AT, Tokmakidis SP. Land versus water exercise in patients with coronary artery disease: Effects on body composition, blood lipids, and physical fitness. Am Heart J 154(3):560, 2007.
8. Meyer K, Steiner R, Lastayo P, et al. Eccentric exercise in coronary patients: Central hemodynamic and metabolic responses. Med Sci Sports Exerc 35(7):1076-1082, 2003.

CUSHING SYNDROME

Overview of Cushing Syndrome

This condition results from excessive levels of cortisol, usually due to adrenocortical tumors or high doses of hydrocortisone or cortisol-derivative drugs. Excessive cortisol results in numerous physiological responses, which include muscle weakness, bone demineralization, weakening of elastic tissues, hyperglycemia, and obesity. Removal of adrenocortical tumors will reverse this syndrome, but patients who rely on hydrocortisone to control their inflammatory disease processes may be unable to reverse this syndrome completely. Removal of the tumor may affect other pituitary hormones, especially growth hormone.[1] The loss of muscle tissues will greatly affect tolerance for daily activities and lead to deconditioning with impaired endurance.

Comorbidities to Consider

• Excessive cortisol affects the cardiac, renal and endocrine systems and contributes to limited activity tolerance.

Client Examination

Keys to Examination of Clients

• Clients are assessed for levels of cortisol in the urine and blood serum.
• Imaging tests visualize the size and position of an adrenocortical tumor.
• Determine the client's weight and body composition before starting an exercise program.
• Bone mineral density tests are useful for clients who have osteopenia.

Recommended Baseline Testing of Fitness Levels

• Use a walking test for the client's exercise tolerance and aerobic capacity.
• Assess the client's muscle strength for large muscle groups with 1- or 10-repetition maximum testing.

Exercise Prescription

Type: Walking, cycling, aquatic exercise[2]
Intensity: Moderate intensities, starting at 40%–60% of maximum Vo_2
Duration: 30 minutes
Frequency: Five times per week

Getting Started

Along with a formal exercise program, clients should be encouraged to increase their daily activity level to increase their daily caloric output.[3] Clients receiving ongoing treatment should avoid exercises that place increased stresses on the skeletal bone and joint structures or that increase the risk of falling. Clients may try other types of exercise as they develop increased strength and have less body fat. Weight lifting and running and stepping activities should be avoided if the cortisol levels are not controlled. Clients with controlled levels of cortisol can be encouraged to do weight-bearing activities to improve bone mineral densities.[2] Weight-bearing exercises should begin at low levels, with 15 to 20 repetitions, with caution to not overload joint structures. Clients can slowly increase the duration of their aerobic activities for up to 60 to 90 minutes. Exercise intensities can slowly progress up to 80% of maximum heart as the client improves aerobic capacity and decreases body weight.[3] A variety of aerobic and resistive exercises can be combined to optimize the client's physical and mental health.

References

1. Cushing's Support and Research Foundation. http://www.csrf.net/page/growth_hormone_deficiency_after_cushings_disease.php. Accessed May 29, 2009.
2. Cushing's Support and Research Foundation. http://www.csrf.net/list/doctors_answers.php. Accessed May 29, 2009.
3. Haskell WL, Lee IM, Pate RR, et al. Physical activity and public health: Updated recommendation for adults from the American College of Sports Medicine and the American Heart Association. Med Sci Sports Exerc 39(8):1423-1434, 2007.

DEPRESSION

Overview of Depression

This condition is a mood disorder characterized by extreme sadness, gloominess, or a sense of melancholy that is frequently associated with physical injury or chronic diseases. Clients may present with persistent muscle and joint pain that is part of a depressive mood disorder. Clients with a history of trauma, low back pain, and systemic diseases are at an increased risk for developing depressive disorders.[1] Depression develops from biochemical and neuroendocrine mechanisms as well as from sleep and psychosocial factors. Depression can be classified as a major depressive disorder, an organic mood disorder, or a bipolar illness. Clients with depression may also suffer from chronic pain, physical impairments, and disease processes, which interfere with daily activities and preclude them from participating in recreational activities. Aerobic endurance activities at moderate intensities have been found to be effective for clients with major depressive disorder of mild to moderate severity.[2]

Comorbidities to Consider

- Chemical dependency is a frequent comorbidity of depression that affects an individual's ability to change behaviors.
- Clients with a history of diseases that affect the cardiovascular and musculoskeletal systems may have limited capacity to improve their endurance and reverse the effects of their disease.

Conditions That May Limit Physical Activities in Clients With Depression

Coronary artery disease	Heart failure
Parkinson disease	Cerebral vascular accident
Diabetes mellitus	Infections
Fibromyalgia	Chronic fatigue syndrome
Arthritis	Cancer treatments

Client Examination

Keys to Examination of Clients

- Screen clients for cardiovascular and musculoskeletal problems that may limit or restrict their participation in an exercise program.
- Assess clients' readiness to begin an exercise program.[3]

Recommended Baseline Testing of Fitness Levels

- Assess baseline aerobic fitness with a 6-minute walk test to assess their progress.
- The Hamilton Rating Scale for Depression can be used as a baseline measurement for depression.[4]

Exercise Prescription

Type: Walking, cycling, recreational pursuits
Intensity: Low to moderate intensity using their perceived exertion
Duration: 15–30 minutes
Frequency: 3–5 days per week

Getting Started

Clients should choose other recreational activities, especially group activities, as these will help them develop regular exercise behaviors.[3,5,6] Strength training can be a useful form of exercise, beginning with low intensities, using multiple sets of 12 to 15 repetitions. A circuit of upper- and lower-extremity exercises is optimal for improving overall strength and endurance while providing the benefits of exercise for depression. A circuit of high-intensity exercise at 80% of maximum, using three sets of eight repetitions, has been shown to decrease depression levels in elderly persons.[7] Clients should be encouraged to try different forms of aerobic activities and recreational pursuits to allow them to maintain a regular exercise program.

References

1. Haggmann S. Screening for symptoms of depression by physical therapist managing low back pain. Phys Ther 84(12):1157-1166, 2004.
2. Dunn AL, Trivedi MH, Kampert JB, et al. Exercise treatment for depression: Efficacy and dose response. Am J Prev Med 28(1):1-8, 2005.
3. Sjösten N, Kivelä SL. The effects of physical exercise on depressive symptoms among the aged: A systematic review. Int J Geriatr Psychiatry 21(5):410-418, 2006.
4. Hamilton Rating Scale for Depression. http://healthnet.umassmed.edu/mhealth/HAMD.pdf. Accessed November 24, 2009.
5. Mead GE, Morley W, Campbell P, et al. Exercise for depression. Cochrane Database Syst Rev 8(3):CD004366, 2009.
6. Blake H, Mo P, Malik S, et al. How effective are physical activity interventions for alleviating depressive symptoms in older people? A systematic review. Clin Rehabil 23(10):873-887, 2009.
7. Singh NA, Stavrinos TM, Scarbek Y, et al. A randomized controlled trial of high- versus low-intensity weight training versus general practitioner care for clinical depression in older adults. J Gerontol A Biol Sci Med Sci 60(6):768-776, 2005.

DIABETES INSIPIDUS

Overview of Diabetes Insipidus

This condition is an imbalance of water due to a deficiency of anti-diuretic hormone (ADH) secreted from the pituitary gland or from insensitivity of the kidneys to ADH. Conditions that affect the posterior pituitary gland and the neurohypophyseal tract limit the secretion of ADH. This condition leads to the excretion of large amounts of diluted urine. Individuals with this condition may become dehydrated, leading to fatigue and irritability.[1] This condition is not related to diabetes mellitus, which affects insulin levels. The deficiency of or insensitivity to ADH does not directly affect an individual's endurance or cardiovascular response to exercise.

Comorbidities to Consider

- Dehydration and polyuria may affect the individual's ability to carry out an effective exercise program.

Client Examination

Keys to Examination of Clients

- Ask clients about test results for ADH levels, urine volume, urine concentrations of water to solutes, and tests of blood plasma concentrations.
- Closely monitor hydration levels before, during, and after exercise.
- Ask clients if they take the medication desmopressin, which is an artificial form of ADH.

Recommended Baseline Testing of Fitness Levels

- Assess for aerobic capacity using walking, running, or cycle ergometer tests.
- Determine if other assessments for muscle strength, body fat measures, and risk for heart disease are needed.

Exercise Prescription

Type: Variety of aerobic and recreational activities
Intensity: Moderate to high intensities
Duration: 30–50 minutes
Frequency: Five to seven times per week

Getting Started

Clients are not restricted in the type of exercise they choose as long as they maintain their hydration. Low-sodium diets help control hydration levels. Exercise programs need to include access to hydration and restrooms. Resistive exercises performed twice per week, using 8 to 12 repetitions that produce a volitional fatigue, are recommended for adults.[2] Clients should be encouraged to maintain a regular exercise program and a healthy lifestyle throughout their life span.[3]

References

1. National Diabetes Insipidus Foundation. http://www.ndif.org/pages/6-Diagnosis__Treatment. Accessed May 26, 2009.
2. Haskell WL, Lee IM, Pate RR, et al. Physical activity and public health: Updated recommendation for adults from the American College of Sports Medicine and the American Heart Association. Med Sci Sports Exerc 39(8):1423-1434, 2007.
3. Diabetes Insipidus Foundation. http://www.diabetesinsipidus.org/4di_gear_up_for_sports.htm. Accessed May 26, 2009.

DIABETES MELLITUS, TYPE 1

Overview of Diabetes Mellitus, Type 1

This condition is due to an autoimmune destruction of the insulin-secreting beta cells of the pancreas. This destruction can be rapid, resulting in this condition presenting in childhood or developing slowly with an initial presentation during early adulthood. The condition results in insufficient levels of insulin to transport glucose into cells, which leads to utilization of fats and proteins as sources of energy, causing severe weight loss and fatigue. Excessive metabolism of fats results in a state of ketoacidosis that can become life-threatening. Clients need ongoing assessment of their blood glucose levels to ensure tight control is maintained, with a proper balance of exogenous insulin, food intake, and exercise.[1] Those who do not control their insulin levels will have limited endurance and develop severe fatigue from increased ketones in the blood stream. Children with this condition who do not have adequate control of their food intake and insulin levels may restrict their physical activities to prevent episodes of ketoacidosis and other complications. Long-term control of hyperglycemia is assessed by the percentage of glycated hemoglobin known as the A_1C test.

Criteria for Tight Diabetes Control

Insulin levels kept between 70 and 130 mg/dL before meals.
Insulin levels at less than 180 mg/dL 2 hours after starting a meal.
A_1C level less than7%.
Use of an insulin pump or multiple injections of insulin per day.

Comorbidities to Consider

- Risk of atherosclerosis, retinopathy, neuropathy, and kidney disease

Client Examination

Keys to Examination of Clients

- Discuss with these clients how to control their blood glucose levels and how to schedule their insulin dosages during the day with an exercise program.
- Clients with previous hypoglycemic episodes are at greater risk for having uncontrolled drops in blood glucose levels, which may be exacerbated with exercise activities.[2]
- Exercise and exercise testing are contraindicated when a client's blood glucose level is greater than 300 mg/dL.
- Screen clients for signs of hypertension, blurred vision, and poor balance before starting an exercise program.

Recommended Baseline Testing of Fitness Levels

- Treadmill or cycle ergometer exercise test or a 6-minute walk or run test can be used to assess aerobic fitness.
- Assess the strength of large-muscle groups with weight-lifting and fitness equipment.
- For clients with no previous exercise experience, you will need to address with them their preparedness and self-efficacy for starting and maintaining a regular exercise program.[3,4]

Exercise Prescription

Type: Aerobic, aquatic, and recreational activities
Intensity: Moderate
Duration: 30–45 minutes
Frequency: Four to five times per week.

Getting Started

Encourage adult clients with type 1 diabetes mellitus to choose a variety of aerobic activities that fit their schedule and lifestyle.[5] Clients may choose aquatic activities, but activities in a warm pool will advance the absorption of injected insulin from superficial tissues, which will require clients to monitor their exercise tolerance more closely. Young clients should be encouraged to participate in a variety of recreational activities for their physical and social benefits.[3]

Adult clients who have difficulties controlling their insulin levels will need to start with a monitored exercise program to determine the effects of exercise on their insulin levels. Make sure the client, when beginning the exercise program, is able to perform and record an assessment of blood glucose levels before and after the exercise session. Ensure the exercise sessions coincide with daily food intake and dosing schedule of exogenous insulin.[2] Adolescent clients should be encouraged to participate in at least 30 minutes of activities each day to prevent cardiovascular disease and to promote an active lifestyle into adulthood.[3] Clients wishing to participate in more endurance training and competitions will need to plan for fluid and carbohydrate intake and assessment of blood glucose levels during their training session. Clients may need to consult with a nutrition expert to properly increase their daily intake of carbohydrates as they increase their training intensities and prepare for competitions.

References

1. American Diabetes Association. http://www.diabetes.org/living-with-diabetes/treatment-and-care/blood-glucose-control/tight-diabetes-control.html. Accessed February 22, 2010.
2. Briscoe VJ, Tate DB, Davis SN. Type 1 diabetes: Exercise and hypoglycemia. Appl Physiol Nutr Metab 32(3):576-582, 2007.
3. Riddell MC, Iscoe KE. Physical activity, sport and pediatric diabetes. Pedatric Diabetes 7:60-70, 2006.
4. Rachmiel M, Buccino J, Daneman D. Exercise and type 1 diabetes mellitus in youth: Review and recommendations. Pediatr Endocrinol Rev 5(2):656-665, 2007.
5. Weltman NY, Saliba SA, Barrett EJ, et al. The use of exercise in the management of type 1 and type 2 diabetes. Clin Sports Med 28:423-439, 2009.

DIABETES MELLITUS, TYPE 2

Overview of Diabetes Mellitus, Type 2

This condition is due to cellular resistance to insulin and deficient insulin secretion, which results in a state of hyperglycemia. A fasting blood glucose level of >126 mg/dL indicates diabetes, with levels of 100 to 125 mg/dL possibly indicating a state of prediabetes.[1] Age, obesity, and a sedentary lifestyle are the main risk factors for developing type 2 diabetes mellitus. The risk of atherosclerosis leading to cardiovascular and peripheral vascular disease is increased in this population, with long-term complications that include kidney damage, retinopathies, and neuropathies. The lack of physical activity is a key risk factor for these clients and is closely linked to their becoming deconditioned, overweight, or obese.[2] This lack of physical activity diminishes clients' skeletal muscle ability to use glucose, and clients become more susceptible to chronic inflammatory conditions that will limit their mobility. Long-term control of hyperglycemia is assessed by the percentage of glycated hemoglobin, known as the A_1C test. Hemoglobin A_1C percentages should be assessed at least twice per year to determine the client's disease status.

Benefits of Exercise for Clients With Type 2 Diabetes Mellitus

Better glycemic control
Improved body composition due to reduced visceral fat and increased muscle tissue
Reduced hyperlipidemia and hypertension
Changes to vascular endothelial lining and improved stroke volume
Reduced development and advancement of cardiovascular diseases

Comorbidities to Consider

- Risk of atherosclerosis leading to cardiovascular and peripheral vascular disease is increased in this population, with long-term complications that include kidney damage, retinopathies, and neuropathies.

Client Examination

Keys to Examination of Clients

- Discuss how well they are able to control their insulin levels and the type and scheduling of medications they use to control their insulin level.
- Screen their overall mobility, vision deficits, and standing balance before starting an exercise program.
- Inspect their shoes and feet to ensure proper support and health of the skin and nails.
- Assess vital signs and circulation in the extremities to determine signs of coronary artery and peripheral vascular diseases.
- Clients with an autonomic neuropathy may have significant increases or decreases of blood pressure with physical activities and are at increased risk for adverse cardiovascular events during exercise.[2]

Simmes Wienstien

Recommended Baseline Testing of Fitness Levels

- Exercise tolerance can be assessed with a graded exercise test using a treadmill or cycle ergometer or the 6-minute walk test.
- Strength of large muscle groups can be assessed with weight-lifting or resistive exercises using 1- or 10-repetition maximums.
- Assess client's self-efficacy before and during exercise programs to promote progression to an independently maintained program.[3]

Exercise Prescription

Type: Aerobic, aquatic, resistive, and recreational activities
Intensity: 60% of maximum heart rate, progressing to 85%
Duration: Up to 50 minutes per day
Frequency: Progress to a goal of three to seven times per week

Getting Started

Consult with your client to identify a number of aerobic and resistive exercises to be used to improve control of glucose levels and improve physical fitness.[4,5] Walking, treadmill walking, elliptical steppers, cycle ergometers, and rowing machines have been used successfully for aerobic exercise.[5-7] Resistive exercises for large-muscle groups can use hand weights or resistive exercise machine that allow the client to make small increases for the intensity of the exercise.[8] Due to the risk of complications from poor thermoregulation, exercising in extreme heat or cold environments should be undertaken with precautions for hydration and protecting the extremities. Clients need to monitor their food and fluid intake before exercising to ensure enough blood glucose is available for their exercise session. Clients using insulin therapy need to assess insulin levels before and during their exercise sessions.

Clients can learn to use their rate of perceived exertion to a level of "somewhat hard" to maintain this level of exercise intensity. Because skeletal muscles are important tissues for glucose utilization, resistive exercise is recommended for glucose control.[9] Design a resistive exercise program that uses moderate to high intensity levels to produce muscle hypertrophy. Exercises using two to four sets of 8 to 10 repetitions, with 1–3 minutes of rest between sets, are recommended for improving muscle strength and increasing muscle tissues. When clients can complete four sets of 8 to 10 repetitions, increase their resistance from 5 to 10 pounds at the next exercise session. Resistive exercise training can be performed three to four times per week.[10] You may choose to prescribe exercises that produce eccentric muscle contractions of the thigh muscles to increase thigh muscle tissue.[5] Provide guidance to your clients to develop regular exercise behaviors at parameters that will sustain glucose control and have other significant health benefits. Consult with other health-care providers to develop long-term programs for clients with type 2 diabetes mellitus that combine components of lifestyle counseling, diet, medications, and exercise.

References

1. Executive summary: Standards of medical care in diabetes—2009. Diabetes Care 32(Suppl 1):S6-S12, 2009.
2. Sigal RJ, Kenny GP, Wasserman DH, et al. Physical activity/exercise and type 2 diabetes: A consensus statement from the American Diabetes Association. Diabetes Care 29(6):1433-1438, 2006.
3. Korkiakangas EE, Alahuhta MA, Laitinen JH. Barriers to regular exercise among adults at high risk or diagnosed with type 2 diabetes: A systematic review. Health Promotion Int 24(4):416-427, 2009.
4. Thomas DE, Elliott EJ, Naughton GA. Exercise for type 2 diabetes mellitus. Cochrane Database Syst Rev 3:CD002968, 2006
5. Marcus RL, Smith S, Morrell G, et al. Comparison of combined aerobic and high-force eccentric resistance exercise with aerobic exercise only for people with type 2 diabetes mellitus. Phys Ther 88(11):1345-1354, 2008.
6. Di Loreto C, Fanelli C, Lucidi P, et al. Make your diabetic patients walk: Long-term impact of different amounts of physical activity on type 2 diabetes. Diabetes Care 28(6):1295-1302, 2005.
7. Araiza P, Hewes H, Gashetewa C. Efficacy of a pedometer-based physical activity program on parameters of diabetes control in type 2 diabetes mellitus. Metabolism 55(10):1382-1387, 2006.
8. Praet SF, van Loon LJ. Exercise therapy in type 2 diabetes. Acta Diabetol 46(4):263-278, 2009.
9. Weltman NY, Saliba SA, Barrett EJ, et al. The use of exercise in the management of type 1 and type 2 diabetes. Clin Sports Med 28: 423-439, 2009.
10. Taylor JD, Fletcher JP, Tiarks J. Impact of physical therapist–directed exercise counseling combined with fitness center–based exercise training on muscular strength and exercise capacity in people with type 2 diabetes: A randomized clinical trial. Phys Ther 89(9):884-892, 2009.

EATING DISORDERS

Overview of Eating Disorders

Eating disorders include anorexia nervosa, bulimia, and binge eating.[1] A combination of genetic, psychological, and social factors results in these disorders. Diminished nutrition, body weight, and muscle mass contribute to endurance impairments. Some clients develop an obsession with exercise in order to limit body weight, which in the long term is not beneficial for their health.[2] Clients may have proximal muscle weakness, which can result in gait disturbances and limitations in performing daily activities. Limitations in endurance must be evaluated within the overall presentations of each client's condition.

Comorbidities to Consider

- Complications for the cardiac, endocrine, and gastrointestinal systems occur owing to altered hydration and electrolyte levels.

Client Examination

Keys to Examination of Clients

- Ask clients if they have been assessed for cardiopulmonary complications and blood and plasma levels.
- Clients with long-standing eating disorders may need assessments of bone mineral densities.
- Consider the need for ongoing psychological and behavioral counseling to address unhealthy habits associated with their eating disorder.[3]

Recommended Baseline Testing of Fitness Levels

- Clients can be assessed for their endurance tolerance, proximal muscle strength, flexibility, and posture.
- Determine the client's beliefs and attitudes about exercise to provide parameters and the types of reinforcement the client will need to maintain the program.

Exercise Prescription

Type: Combine aerobic activities with resistive exercise and relaxation methods
Intensity: Low to moderate intensities using heart rate and perceived exertion levels
Duration: Start at 15–30 minutes
Frequency: Three to five times per week

Getting Started

The initial exercise program will need to be carefully planned and supervised to ensure the client's adherence to a cognitive behavioral therapy program. Clients will need to adhere to nutritional and behavioral standards in order to participate in an exercise program. A combination of aerobic activities, resistive exercises, stretching, and relaxation methods will provide a balanced approach to exercise with an emphasis on lifelong fitness and promotion of positive body image.[4] Clients who have developed excessive exercise habits will need to have specific upper limits on their program.[5] Clients with cardiopulmonary complications will need ongoing assessment of heart rate and blood pressure to ensure exercise is performed within a prescribed intensity level.

A written record of exercise will help clients develop an understanding of their abilities and self-confidence.[5] Aerobic exercises can be performed at 50% to 70% of clients' maximum heart rate for up to 45 minutes.[4] Use of a treadmill, cycle ergometer, or elliptical trainer is recommended to help clients record and provide feedback on their parameters of exercise.[6] Resistive exercises can be performed at moderate intensities, with an emphasis on maintaining good postures and exercise form. Clients will need to monitor symptoms of fatigue and pain in order to self-limit exercise intensities and durations.

Clients should be encouraged frequently with reinforcement of their gains in exercise abilities. Exercise programs can be advanced if the client believes the program is relaxing and rejuvenating. Clients experiencing fatigue or excessive anxiety about their program need to have their program re-evaluated. Clients who demonstrate adherence to their exercise program and parameters should be encouraged to exercise in a group or social setting.[6]

References

1. National Eating Disorders Association. http://www.nationaleatingdisorders.org/information-resources/general-information.php. Accessed July 9, 2009.
2. Mond JM, Hay PJ, Rodgers B, et al. An update on the definition of "excessive exercise" in eating disorders research. Int J Eating Disorders 39(2):147-153, 2006.
3. Calogero RM, Pedrotty KN. The practice and process of healthy exercise: An investigation of the treatment of exercise abuse in women with eating disorders. Eating Disorders 12(4):273-291, 2004.
4. Hausenblas HA, Cook BJ, Chittester NI. Can exercise treat eating disorders? Exerc Sport Sci Rev. 36(1):43-47, 2008.
5. Beumont PJ, Arthur B, Russell JD, et al. Excessive physical activity in dieting disorder patients: Proposals for a supervised exercise program. Int J Eating Disorders 15(1):21-36, 1994.
6. Sundgot-Borgen J, Rosenvinge J. Bahr R, et al. The effect of exercise, cognitive therapy, and nutritional counseling in treating bulimia nervosa. Med Sci Sports Exerc 34(2):190-195, 2002.

EPILEPSY

Overview of Epilepsy

This condition is a chronic disorder characterized by recurrent seizures. The seizures can be partial or generalized, depending on the extent that the brain is affected by abnormal electrical activity. There are numerous causes for seizures, but the majority of epilepsy cases are idiopathic. Epilepsy does not directly produce endurance impairments, but the secondary effects and medications are associated with decreased physical activities. The effect of exercise as a positive or negative influence on seizure frequency in unknown.[1] Individuals, especially children, avoid physical and group activities that may be dangerous or embarrassing if a seizure occurs.[2,3]

Comorbidities to Consider

• Clients with symptomatic epilepsy may have neurologic conditions that significantly affect their mobility and ability to participate in exercise activities.

Client Examination

Keys to Examination of Clients

• An electroencephalogram helps with the diagnosis and classification of epilepsy.
• Determine if clients have mobility limitations or a history of physical conditions.
• Discuss with clients their beliefs about and experience with physical activities.

Recommended Baseline Testing of Fitness Levels

• Aerobic capacity can be assessed with submaximal tests using walking and cycle ergometry.
• Develop baseline assessments of posture, balance, and flexibility before prescribing an exercise program.

Exercise Prescription

Type: Walking, bicycling, weight training, swimming
Intensity: Moderate to high levels
Duration: 30–50 minutes
Frequency: Three to four times per week

Getting Started

Individuals with epilepsy can participate in most modes of exercise, as a seizure induced by exercise is relatively uncommon.[1] Because individuals with epilepsy have been found to have fitness levels below normal levels, aerobic training for the benefit of cardiovascular health and weight control is commonly advised for these individuals. Individuals with epilepsy are advised to avoid extreme environmental conditions, which may be dangerous in the event of a seizure. Exercising in high temperature and high humidity should be avoided, as hyperthermia has been associated with the onset of seizure. Resistance training along with a variety of recreational activities to improve fitness can be utilized.[2] Participation in contact sports or sports with the potential for collisions should be cleared by a client's physician. After a seizure event, individuals may be advised to avoid physical exertions for a period of a few weeks. Clients should be encouraged to try different types of exercise to develop lifelong exercise behaviors.

References

1. Arida RM, Cavalheiro EA, daSilva AC, et al. Physical activity and epilepsy. Sports Med 38(7):607-615, 2008.
2. Wong J, Wirrell E. Physical activity in children/teens with epilepsy compared with that in their siblings without epilepsy. Epilepsia 47(3):631-639, 2006.
3. Nakken KO. Physical exercise in outpatients with epilepsy. Epilepsia 40(5):643-651, 1999.

FIBROMYALGIA

Overview of Fibromyalgia

This condition is considered a syndrome of chronic muscle pain associated with a neuro-hormonal dysfunction of the autonomic nervous system. Individuals with this systemic condition have widespread tender or trigger points and may have symptoms associated with chronic fatigue syndrome.[1] Individuals are diagnosed by a process of elimination and may require multiple tests of endocrine and immunity systems to rule out other disorders. These individuals commonly receive treatment for depression, which may also benefit from an exercise program.[2] However, they find many activities difficult to perform due to diffuse, persistent pain. Individuals limit their activities in an effort to decrease or control their ongoing symptoms.

Benefits of an Exercise Program for a Client With Fibromyalgia

Increased levels of endorphins
Increased metabolic rate
Improved sleep patterns

Increased cortisol levels
Increased lean-tissue mass
Decreased pain and fatigue

Comorbidities to Consider

• Depression and other mood disorders are commonly found.

Client Examination

Keys to Examination of Clients

• Perform baseline testing of clients' mobility, posture, and flexibility before prescribing an exercise program.
• Discuss with clients their beliefs and experience with exercise, as they may be reluctant to start an exercise program. Discuss with them the likelihood that increasing levels of activities will be associated with increased pain severity and fatigue.

Recommended Baseline Testing of Fitness Levels

• Use the 6-minute walk test as a recommended baseline of aerobic fitness and tolerance to exercise.[3]
• Employ the global pain rating scale, tender point count, and the Fibromyalgia Impact Questionnaire to establish a baseline of muscle pain symptoms.[2,4]

Exercise Prescription

Type: Aerobic activities, aquatic therapies, weight training
Intensity: Begin with very low levels
Duration: Short bouts of 2–5 minutes, with rest periods
Frequency: Three to four times per week

Getting Started

Aerobic exercise is considered the most important element of an exercise program for individuals with fibromyalgia, but strengthening exercises have also been found to have similar effects for changes in physical and psychological parameters.[5-7] Aerobic exercises should be started at levels just below clients' capacity, and progressions should be gradual. Individuals may need to start with 2- to 5-minute bouts at low intensities. Aquatic exercise in warm pools (>85°F) is a highly recommended form of exercise.[2] Individuals will find muscle-stretching routines and movement therapies, such as t'ai chi and Pilates, a good start to a regular exercise program.[3,8] Progressing intensities to 60% to 75% of age-adjusted maximum heart rate is recommended, but clients should be taught perceived exertion methods for determining the intensity of their exercise programs.[3,9] Group exercise should be avoided initially until clients are able to self-control their level of intensity and can maintain exercise for longer periods.[2] Strengthening exercise can be in many forms, such as free weights, pulley systems, or body weight, starting with minimal resistance and five or six repetitions. These exercises should avoid excessive eccentric muscle contractions initially to delay onset of muscle soreness.[5,6] Slow increases in the intensity and duration of exercise are needed along with the clients' self-efficacy for believing they are ready to progress their exercise intensity.

References

1. Wolfe F, Smythe HA, Yunus MB, et al. The American College of Rheumatology 1990 criteria for the classification of fibromyalgia: Report of the multicenter criteria committee. Arthritis Rheum 33:160-172, 1990.
2. Gowans SE, deHueck A. Exercise for fibromyalgia: Benefits and practical advice. J Musculoskeletal Med 22:614-622, 2006.
3. Gowans SE, deHueck A. Pool exercise for individuals with fibromyalgia. Curr Opin Rheumatol 19(2): 168-173, 2007.
4. Fibromyalgia Impact Questionnaire. www.myalgia.com/FIQ/fiq.pdf. Accessed November 24, 2009.
5. Busch AJ, Schachter CL, Overend TJ, et al. Exercise for fibromyalgia: A systematic review. J Rheumatol 35(6):1130-1144, 2008.
6. Bircan C, Karasel SA, Akgün B. Effects of muscle strengthening versus aerobic exercise program in fibromyalgia. Rheumatol Int 28(6):527-532, 2008.
7. Brosseau L, Wells GA, Tugwell P, et al. Ottawa Panel evidence-based clinical practice guidelines for aerobic fitness exercises in the management of fibromyalgia: Part 1. Phys Ther 88(7): 857-871, 2008.
8. Altan L, Korkmaz N, Bingol U, et al. Effect of Pilates training on people with fibromyalgia syndrome: A pilot study. Arch Phys Med Rehabil 90(12):1983-1988, 2009.
9. Gowans SE, Dehueck A, Voss S, et al. Six-month and one-year follow-up of 23 weeks of aerobic exercise for individuals with fibromyalgia. Arthritis Rheum 51(6):890-898, 2004.

HEMOPHILIA

Overview of Hemophilia

Hemophilia is a bleeding disorder caused by abnormal plasma-clotting proteins. Clients with hemophilia have prolonged bleeding times and the risk of internal hemorrhaging into joints and muscles. This disorder is classified by the client's percentage of clotting factors: mild is 5% to 50%; moderate is 1% to 5%; severe is <1%. Patients with moderate and severe hemophilia will need factor replacement therapy to control and prevent excessive bleeding. Individuals with hemophilia may develop limited endurance from a combination of factors that include repeated joint bleeds, pain and limited joint mobility, muscle atrophy, and fear of injury. Limited endurance is associated with decreased muscle strength, joint stability, and proprioception.[1,2]

Comorbidities to Consider

• Clients may contract hepatitis C from blood transfusions and develop liver disease.

Client Examination

Keys to Examination of Clients

• The stages of joint degeneration secondary to joint bleeds are determined by radiographs of joints using the Arnold-Hilgartner and Pettersson scales.[3]
• Discuss with clients if they have developed "target joints" from repeated bleeding episodes, which will need to be assessed carefully for mobility and signs of synovitis.

Arnold-Hilgartner Criteria for Stages of Hemophilic Arthropathy

0: Normal joint
1: Soft-tissue swelling, no skeletal abnormalities
2: Osteopenia and overgrowth of epiphysis, normal joint space
3: Changes in osseous contours, formation of chondral cysts
4: Narrowing of joint space, signs of articular cartilage destructions
5: Substantial disorganization of joint structures

Recommended Baseline Testing of Fitness Levels

• Aerobic fitness testing can be performed with walking or cycle ergometry methods.[4,5]
• Assess for client risk of falling and the ability to control movements without risking overstressing joints and muscle groups.
• Client may need to take clotting factor replacement therapy before engaging in testing and new exercise programs.[6]

Exercise Prescription

Type: Recreational and fitness activities[4]
Intensity: Moderate intensities, 60%–80% of peak heart rate.
Duration: 30–60 minutes
Frequency: Three to five times per week

Getting Started

Individuals with hemophilia need to choose safe and appropriate activities that will not place them at risk for recurrent joint and muscle bleeds.[4] Young people can be encouraged to participate in recreational and competitive swimming as these activities pose minimal risk for bleeding episodes, provide social interactions, and can be performed for a lifetime.[2] Some young people with hemophilia may rebel against restrictions on their participation in sports and recreational activities.[5]

Resistive exercise should be started at low levels with an emphasis on endurance activities of 15 to 20 repetitions. The client's movements and technique should be closely monitored to ensure good joint stability and control of the motion. The exercises should avoid excessive eccentric muscle loading so as to prevent micro-traumas that could lead to muscle bleeds.[6] Clients may need a referral to a physical therapist after a significant bleed to regain normal motion and to develop a plan for returning to the regular exercise program. [6]

References

1. Gomis M, Querol F, Gallach JE, et al. Exercise and sport in the treatment of haemophilic patients: A systematic review. Haemophilia 15(1):43-54, 2009.
2. Herbsleb M, Hilberg T. Maximal and submaximal endurance performance in adults with severe haemophilia. Haemophilia 15(1):114-121, 2009.
3. Kilcoyne RF, Nuss R. Radiological assessment of haemophilic arthropathy with emphasis on MRI findings. Haemophilia 9(Suppl 1):57-64, 2003.
4. National Hemophilia Foundation. http://www.hemophilia.org/NHFWeb/Resource/StaticPages/menu0/menu5/menu60/menu112/SportsRatingsActivity.pdf. Accessed November 24, 2009.
5. Mulder K, Cassis F, Seuser DR, et al. Risks and benefits of sports and fitness activities for people with haemophilia. Haemophilia 10(Suppl 4):161-163, 2004.
6. Wittmier K, Mulder K. Enhancing lifestyle for individuals with haemophilia through physical activity and exercise: The role of physiotherapy. Haemophilia 13(Suppl 2):31-37, 2007.

HEPATITIS

Overview of Hepatitis

Hepatitis is an inflammation of liver tissues caused by viruses, chemical exposure, drug reaction, or alcohol abuse. Viral hepatitis presents and progresses in various forms. Acute hepatitis results initially in fatigue, nausea, mild fever, and right upper quadrant abdominal discomfort. Chronic hepatitis can lead to end-stage liver failure requiring an organ transplant. Clients with hepatitis may experience fatigue and arthralgia severe enough to limit their normal activities. Acute hepatitis requires the client to conserve energy, but even as the condition begins to resolve, the client may still have significant fatigue.

Comorbidities to Consider

- Chronic hepatitis may produce complications that include neuropathy, arthralgias, and myalgias, with rare occurrences of rheumatic diseases.

Client Examination

Keys to Examination of Clients

- Laboratory testing of blood serum identifies the type of viral hepatitis.
- A liver biopsy determines the stage of the disease.
- Assess for signs of dehydration, edema, fluid weight gain, or respiratory difficulties.

Recommended Baseline Testing of Fitness Levels

- Clients who want to return to their usual exercise and recreational activities should be assessed for their exercise tolerance.
- Screen for balance and coordination to determine if normal neuromuscular function is present.
- Assess for joint mobility and muscle extensibility to determine a loss of mobility.

Exercise Prescription

Type: Aerobic and fitness activities[1]
Intensity: Moderate intensities
Duration: 30 minutes or more
Frequency: Three to five times per week

Getting Started

Clients may choose a variety of individual and group activities for their exercise programs and should be encouraged to use a variety of activities. Exercise intensity can be monitored by heart rate and perceived exertion levels. Clients who have recovered from acute hepatitis may return to their previous activities or sports when they are medically cleared.[2] Clients in the initial or acute phases of hepatitis need to conserve energy and are not able to continue with their normal recreational or athletic activities.[2] Clients should begin slowly and progress as they tolerate longer durations and greater intensities of exercise. As their condition resolves, clients may increase their daily activities and begin a return to their exercise programs. Clients with chronic hepatitis should be encouraged to participate in low- to moderate-level activities, but they should avoid any strenuous or prolonged physical activities.[1,2] A study of individuals receiving treatment for chronic hepatitis C virus found significant improvements in fitness levels and quality of life measures after an 8-month program of aerobic training of 5 days per week.[1]

References

1. Payen JL, Pillard F, Mascarell V, et al. Is physical activity possible and beneficial for patients with hepatitis C receiving pegylated interferon and ribavirin therapy? Gastroenterol Clin Biol 33(1 Pt 1):8-14, 2009.
2. Harrington DW. Viral hepatitis and exercise. Med Sci Sports Exerc 32(7 Suppl):S422-430, 2000.

HYPERTENSION

Overview of Hypertension

Hypertension is characterized by an increase of systolic and/or diastolic blood pressure. The most common type of hypertension is termed primary or idiopathic. Secondary hypertension is associated with numerous diseases, disorders, and traumatic injuries. The National Institutes of Health define hypertension as systolic blood pressure of over 140 or diastolic pressure over 90 mm Hg. Prehypertension is defined as systolic pressure of 120 to 139 or a diastolic pressure of 80 to 89 mm Hg.[1] The most common source of hypertension is from narrowing of the arterioles, which is controlled by the sympathetic nervous system and the rennin-angiotensin system of the kidneys.

Obesity and sedentary lifestyles are major risk factors for developing hypertension. Clients with hypertension experience limited endurance from dyspnea and increased fatigue with activities. Hypertension is controlled by reducing risk factors and drug therapies. Vasodilators comprise a class of drugs that produce peripheral vasodilations, which reduces blood pressure. Beta blockers are drugs that diminish the heart rate response to activities and limit blood pressure and myocardial contractility. Angiotensin-converting enzyme (ACE) inhibitors and calcium channel blockers reduce the peripheral vascular resistance, and diuretic drugs control the volume of blood.

Risk Factors for Hypertension Affected by an Exercise Program

Reduced risk of obesity   Decreased sedentary lifestyle behaviors
Reduced stress levels   Better control of diabetes mellitus

Comorbidities to Consider

• Hypertension affects multiple organs and increases the risk of atherosclerosis, which leads to damage of the heart and brain tissue.

Client Examination

Keys to Examination of Clients

• Clients with hypertension should have their blood counts, blood glucose, serum levels of potassium, and cholesterol levels assessed regularly as well as having electrocardiograms.
• Ask clients about the type and schedule of drug therapies they use for controlling hypertension.
• Perform frequent monitoring of heart rate and blood pressure during and after exercise sessions.

Recommended Baseline Testing of Fitness Levels

• Perform walking or cycle ergometer tests to assess aerobic capacity and exercise tolerance.
• Assess extremity mobility and strength levels before prescribing resistive exercises.

Exercise Prescription

Type: Walking, running, cycling, weight training[2-5]
Intensity: Moderate intensity, starting at 40%-60% of maximum aerobic capacity[2]
Duration: 30 minutes
Frequency: Five times per week

Getting Started

Clients will need at least 10 minutes for warm-up and cool-down during their exercise session. Because different types of drugs are used to control hypertension, the increase in heart rate is not recommended as the sole determinant for measuring the intensity of exercises. Perceived exertion levels are best for grading exercise intensity for clients using calcium channel and beta blockers. Clients should develop exercise habits to increase the duration and frequency of their exercise activities.[4] Clients should not exercise in excessive heat as excessive sweating and vascular dilation affect blood volume and pressure. Indications to stop an exercise session include development of headache, a flush, tingling in the limbs, increased dyspnea, chest pain, and confusion. Resistance training appearance can be used with low intensities and high repetitions to reduce diastolic blood pressures.[3] Heavy resistance exercise and isometric contractions are contraindicated for these individuals due to the risk of increasing blood pressure to harmful levels.

Clients should maintain their exercise program for at least 6 months to have lasting effects on their blood pressure. Regular exercise benefits clients with obesity and other risk factors that are diminished by aerobic exercise. Clients with hypertension participating in athletic activities and recreational sports can exercise at advanced levels by using ACE inhibitors and calcium channel blockers.[2]

References

1. National Heart Lung Blood Institute. http://www.nhlbi.nih.gov/health/dci/Diseases/Hbp/HBP_WhatIs.htm Accessed November 5, 2009.
2. Pescatello LS, Franklin BA, Fagard R, et al. American College of Sports Medicine position stand: Exercise and hypertension. Med Sci Sports Exerc 36(3):533-553, 2004.
3. Fagard RH. Exercise is good for your blood pressure: Effects of endurance training and resistance training. Clin Exp Pharmacol Physiol 33(9):853-856, 2006.
4. Whelton SP, Chin A, Xin X, et al. Effect of aerobic exercise on blood pressure: A meta-analysis of randomized, controlled trials. Ann Intern Med 136(7):493-503, 2002.
5. Calhoun DA, Jones D, Textor S, et al. Resistant hypertension: Diagnosis, evaluation, and treatment. Circulation 117(25):510-526, 2008.

HYPERTHYROIDISM

Overview of Hyperthyroidism

Hyperthyroidism results in generalized elevation of metabolism and increased activity of the sympathetic nervous system. Graves disease is the most common form of hyperthyroidism. Manifestations include weight loss, tremor, heart palpitations, sweating, and heat intolerance. This condition increases the metabolic rate and oxygen consumption, requiring an increased supply of oxygen and removal of metabolic products from the skeletal muscles.[1] Hyperthyroidism may cause an over-reliance on muscle glycogen during exercise programs.[2] Those who develop arthralgias secondary to this condition will greatly reduce their daily activities in order to control joint pains. Severe cases of hyperthyroidism may result in myopathy of the proximal and respiratory muscles. Treatment usually results in insufficient thyroid hormone production, requiring the client to take synthetic thyroid hormone.

Comorbidities to Consider

- Chronic hyperthyroidism can result in periarthritis, myopathy, and reduced cardiac function.

Client Examination

Keys to Examination of Clients

- Clients will have undergone tests for blood levels of thyroid-stimulating hormone, thyroid hormones, and radioactive iodine uptake.
- Carefully assess heart rate and blood pressure as clients may have tachycardia and abnormal systolic and diastolic blood pressures at rest and with exercise.[1]
- Ask clients about medications they use to control the production of thyroid hormones.

Recommended Baseline Testing of Fitness Levels

- Assess aerobic function by means of treadmill or cycle ergometer.
- Assess strength of the proximal muscles through dynamometry and tests of one-repetition maximum.[3]
- Determine body composition for the relationship of lean mass to total body weight.

Exercise Prescription

Type: Walking; weight-training programs.
Intensity: 60%–80% of one-repetition maximum for 8–10 repetitions
Duration: 15–30 minutes
Frequency: Two to three times per week

Getting Started

Individuals with severe hyperthyroidism need a complete resistive exercise program in order to regain normal levels of strength and muscle mass.[3] Individuals with well-controlled cases can participate in exercise and recreational programs of their choice. During exercise activities the client should be regularly assessed for signs of heat intolerance, which may include excessive sweating, muscle cramping, nausea, tingling in the extremities, and syncope. After exercise, a client's heart rate may stay elevated for an extended period. Resistive exercise performed 2 days per week for 16 weeks has been found to result in significant increases in muscle strength and promote muscle mass in clients receiving treatment for hyperthyroidism.[1] Clients with well-controlled conditions should be encouraged to maintain an exercise program three to five times per week for at least 30 minutes to maintain muscle strength and decrease the risk of developing heart disease.[4] Clients with this condition can increase their resistive exercise program if the program does not increase their level of fatigue or heat intolerance and does not bring on joint pain.

References

1. Kahaly GJ, Kampmann C, Mohr-Kahaly S. Cardiovascular hemodynamics and exercise tolerance in thyroid disease. Thyroid 12(6):473-481, 2002.
2. McAllister RM, Delp MD, Laughlin MH. Thyroid status and exercise tolerance: Cardiovascular and metabolic considerations. Sports Med 20(3):189-198, 1995.
3. Bousquet-Santos K, Vaisman M, Barreto ND, et al. Resistance training improves muscle function and body composition in patients with hyperthyroidism. Arch Phys Med Rehabil 87(8):1123-1130, 2006.
4. Merucuro G, Panzuto MG, Bina A, et al. Cardiac function, physical exercise capacity, and quality of life during long-term thyrotropin-suppressive therapy with levotyroxine: Effect of individual dose tailoring. Clin Endocrin Metab 85(1):159-164, 2000.

HYPOTHYROIDISM

Overview of Hypothyroidism

Hypothyroidism is a deficiency of thyroid hormones, due primarily to decreased synthesis or size of the thyroid gland. A deficiency of thyroid hormones affects multiple systems, which can result in slower metabolism, muscle weakness, advanced atherosclerosis, and slower mental functions. Individuals may have a subclinical hypothyroidism even though their thyroid hormone levels are within normal value limits.[1] This condition is reversed with administration of synthetic thyroid hormones. Decreased thyroid hormone levels affect connective tissues of the cardiovascular system, resulting in decreased cardiac output, slowed heart rate, and diminished peripheral circulation.[1,2] Proximal muscle weakness along with complaints of stiffness, muscle pain, and trigger points make daily activities more difficult to complete.

Systemic Manifestations That Affect Exercise Tolerance

Central nervous system: Fatigue and headaches
Cardiovascular system: Heart failure, angina, poor peripheral circulation, dyspnea
Musculoskeletal system: Proximal muscle weakness, myalgia, joint swelling
Gastrointestinal system: Weight gain, decreased absorption of nutrients

Comorbidities to Consider

- Long-term use of synthetic thyroid hormones may lead to limited cardiac functions and exercise tolerances.[3]

Client Examination

Keys to Examination of Clients

- Ask clients about their laboratory tests for their levels of thyroid-stimulating hormones and thyroxine (T_4). Hypothyroidism can significantly elevate serum cholesterol and triglyceride levels.
- Take vital signs, and look for signs of congestive heart failure as clients recently diagnosed with this condition may have atherosclerosis with or without angina. Administration of synthetic hormones increases heart muscle activity, which may aggravate angina symptoms.

Recommended Baseline Testing of Fitness Levels

- Tests of aerobic fitness and muscle strength should begin with very low levels of exertion, with monitoring of clients' symptoms and tolerance to the activities.
- Screen clients for their preparedness to begin an exercise program.

Exercise Prescription

Type: Walking, cycling
Intensity: Low levels; start at 50% of maximum heart rate
Duration: Short bouts, with regular vital sign assessments
Frequency: Five to seven times per week

Getting Started

Aerobic exercises should be chosen to allow long-term adoption of an independent exercise program. Interventions to address myalgia and trigger points may be needed before beginning a regular exercise program. Clients with severe muscle and joint pain may only tolerate interventions to regain motion and increase activity levels. Exercise-induced muscle pain may be a precursor to rhabdomyolysis, which will result in further muscle damage and renal failure. Strengthening activities should also be started at low level of intensities, with an emphasis of higher repetitions (15 to 20) and performing motions through full ranges and proper form. Gradual progression of exercise programs allows clients to improve their exercise tolerance and for tissue adaptations that provide for maintenance of cardiovascular function and muscle strength. Education is important to help clients understand the need for a lifetime commitment to physical activities and exercise of their choosing to prevent the progression of their heart disease.

References

1. Ochs N, Auer R, Bauer DC, et al. Meta-analysis: Subclinical thyroid dysfunction and the risk for coronary heart disease and mortality. Ann Intern Med 148(11):832-845, 2008.
2. Biondi B, Klein I. Hypothyroidism as a risk factor for cardiovascular disease. Endocrine 24(1):1-13, 2004.
3. Salerno M, Oliviero U, Lettiero T, et al. Long-term cardiovascular effects of levothyroxine therapy in young adults with congenital hypothyroidism. J Clin Endocrinol Metab 93(7):2486-2491, 2008.

INFLAMMATORY BOWEL DISEASE (IBD)

Overview of IBD

Crohn disease and ulcerative colitis are two types of inflammatory conditions of the bowel. Crohn disease affects segments of the intestinal tract, characterized by exacerbations and remissions. Ulcerative colitis can affect the entire colon, which produces ongoing problems with diarrhea and bleeding. Both conditions have genetic and immunologic causes, with most occurrences in young adults. Individuals with these conditions may have limited endurance due to ongoing problems with fatigue and malnutrition. Abdominal and joint pain may also limit an individual's ability to participate in regular exercise programs.[1,2] The effects of exercise on the IBD process has not been clearly determined.

Comorbidities to Consider

- These conditions are associated with osteoporosis, arthralgias, and inflammatory conditions, but they are not characterized by a specific form of arthritis.

Client Examination

Keys to Examination of Clients

- These conditions require numerous imaging studies and endoscopies of the abdominal tract.
- Measurements of bone mineral densities are appropriate for clients with ongoing persistent symptoms.[1]

Recommended Baseline Testing of Fitness Levels

- Tests of aerobic fitness using walking or stationary bicycling are the most appropriate methods for assessment.[2]
- Resistive strength testing may also be performed if the client chooses to incorporate resistive exercises in the exercise program.
- Assess for spinal and extremity ranges of motion and muscle length tests for the client with a history of arthralgias or ankylosing spondylitis.

Exercise Prescription

Type: Walking, cycling, weight training[1,3]
Intensity: Start at low intensities or self-paced walking
Duration: 30 minutes
Frequency: Three times per week

Getting Started

Clients with IBD experience periods of exacerbations that will preclude or limit their participation in an exercise program. During exacerbations, clients may need intermittent rest during the day to conserve energy and decrease bowel motility.[1] Clients with IBD may be at risk for overexertion if they overestimate their work capacities.[3] Clients can add other aerobic and resistive exercises as they progress their program. Resistive exercise, especially for the lower extremities, consisting of squatting, stepping, and lunging exercises are useful for improving tolerance to daily activities.[4] Individuals with IBD should be encouraged to participate in low-intensity recreational activities and to increase their exercise durations and frequencies while maintaining low to moderate intensities with aerobic and resistive exercise. Clients who have undergone moderate to extensive resection of the colon will be restricted from any high-intensity exercises.[5]

References

1. Neeraj N, Fedorak RN. Exercise and inflammatory bowel disease. Can J Gastroenterol 22(5):497–504, 2008.
2. Ng V, Millard W, Lebrun C. Exercise and Crohn's disease: Speculations on potential benefits. Can J Gastroenterol 20(10):657-660, 2006.
3. Ng V, Millard W, Lebrun C. Low-intensity exercise improves quality of life in patients with Crohn's disease. Clin J Sport Med 17(5):384-388, 2007.
4. Wiroth JB, Filippi J, Schneider SM, et al. Muscle performance in patients with Crohn's disease in clinical remission. Inflamm Bowel Dis 11(3):296-303, 2005.
5. Brevinge H, Berglund B, Bosaeus I. Exercise capacity in patients undergoing proctocolectomy and small bowel resection for Crohn's disease. Br J Surg 82(8):1040-1045, 1995.

LUPUS, SYSTEMIC ERYTHEMATOSUS (SLE)

Overview of SLE

SLE is a chronic inflammatory autoimmune disorder that can affect any system of the body. The body's production of antibodies suppresses the immune response and damages tissues. Clients with SLE typically present with a history of chronic fatigue, obesity, and ischemic heart disease.[1] They may present with a complex of signs and symptoms that may require numerous medical test to monitor. They may have chronic fatigue and sleep disturbances, causing them to tend to rest, even though pain and weakness do not limit activities. Endurance impairments develop owing to limited activities and changes to the cardiovascular system.[1] Renal problems can result in hypertension and edema in the extremities.

Comorbidities to Consider

- Clients may develop cardiovascular conditions, arthralgias, neuropathies, and chronic fatigue.

Client Examination

Keys to Examination of Clients

- Regularly assess heart rate, blood pressure, and respiratory rate when starting clients on an exercise program.

Recommended Baseline Testing of Fitness Levels

- Use a walking test to assess aerobic capacity tests.
- Measure fatigue by using the Fatigue Severity Score or a visual analog scale.[2]

Exercise Prescription

Type: Walking, treadmill walking, stationary cycling, and swimming[1,3]
Intensity: Start at low intensities
Duration: 20–30 minutes
Frequency: Three times per week

Getting Started

Aerobic exercises can be progressed by increasing the duration of the treatment sessions as this will help improve the client's tolerance to exercise activities and can result in improved tolerance to more daily activities.[1] Clients with severe manifestations or flare-ups of SLE will need to pace activities to conserve energy and may be unable to maintain a consistent exercise program. Clients with SLE may have photosensitivities that may limit or preclude exercise programs outdoors. Clients with neuropsychiatric manifestations should be monitored for cognitive dysfunctions and may need precautions for seizures. Aerobic activities at 70% to 80% of maximum heart rate for 30 to 40 minutes three times a week have been shown to result in a significant improvement in aerobic capacity, exercise tolerance, and quality-of-life measurements.[4] A heart rate monitor is recommended to ensure the client is maintaining an adequate intensity of exercise. Swimming or water exercises require periodic checks of heart rate levels to ensure an adequate intensity of exercise. Resistance exercises can be performed with low weights with two to three sets of 12 repetitions using muscle groups whose weakness is limiting daily activities.

References

1. Ayan C, Martin V. Systemic lupus erythematosus and exercise. Lupus 16:5-9, 2007.
2. Tench CM, McCarthy J, McCurdie I, et al. Fatigue in systemic lupus erythematosus: A randomized controlled trial of exercise. Rheumatology (Oxford) 42(9):1050-1054, 2003.
3. Strömbeck B, Jacobsson LT.The role of exercise in the rehabilitation of patients with systemic lupus erythematosus and patients with primary Sjögren's syndrome. Curr Opin Rheumatol 19(2):197-203, 2007.
4. Carvalho MR, Sato EI, Tebexreni AS, et al. Effects of supervised cardiovascular training program on exercise tolerance, aerobic capacity, and quality of life in patient with systemic lupus erythematosus. Arthritis Rheum 53(6):838-844, 2005.

LYMPHEDEMA

Overview of Lymphedema

This condition is usually caused by decreased capacity of the lymphatic system to maintain normal flow of lymphatic fluids. The most common causes of lymphedema are invasive procedures and surgical resection of tissues for the treatment of cancer. Severity progresses in three stages (see following). Clients with this condition are unable to use their affected extremities in a normal manner, limiting their daily activities and ability to participate in recreational activities.[1] Clients with advanced stages of lymphedema will need a comprehensive treatment program to manage their condition.

Stages of Lymphedema

Stage I: Development of pitting edema in extremities, which is reversible on elevation of the limb.

Stage II: Irreversible edema with development of connective tissue fibrosis.

Stage III: Severe fibrotic edema with atrophic changes throughout the affected extremity.

Comorbidities to Consider

- Clients who have developed this condition secondary to treatment of cancer may have severe fatigue that limits their activity level.

Client Examination

Keys to Examination of Clients

- Limb volume can be measured with circumferential measurements or by water volumetry.
- Heart rate and blood pressure are important in assessing the effects of changes in fluid levels upon the cardiovascular system.
- Clients may have undergone imaging studies to determine if other causes of limited lymphatic flow are present or a lymphoscintigraphy to measure peripheral lymphatic function using radiotracers.
- Examine for signs of skin breakdown as repetitive movements may cause stress to the skin.

Recommended Baseline Testing of Fitness Levels

- Exercise tolerance can be assessed with an arm ergometer test or with a walking test of short durations.
- Strength assessment of the involved limb will be difficult as the client may be unable to support the limb independently, and excessive pressure on the limb should be avoided.

Exercise Prescription

Type: Walking, arm ergometry, weight training[2-4]
Intensity: Start with low intensities
Duration: Start with short bouts with rest periods
Frequency: Three to five times per week

Getting Started

The exercise program needs to be coordinated with other aspects of the client's medical management. Clients who have undergone treatment for cancer, especially after mastectomy, may be counseled to limit the use of their involved upper extremity and may fear that overusing their involved extremity will worsen their condition. Exercise has the potential to have negative effects on the client's condition and should be carefully prescribed and monitored. Recommended programs for clients with upper-extremity lymphedema include a supervised circuit of weight training exercises for the upper and lower extremities along with an aerobic component using arm ergometry.[1-6] Clients may need to wear a compression sleeve during their exercise program if they are receiving other types of treatment for their condition.[7] Exercise programs for clients with lower extremity lymphedema have not been described.

Upper extremity exercises, using hand weights, starting with 0.5 to 1 pound, are recommended. Exercise programs typically progress to moderate intensities using hand weights and variable resistance equipment for the upper and lower extremities with three sets of 10 repetitions.[3,4,6,7] The suggested sequence of activities begins with proximal muscle groups followed by movements of the distal extremities. Aerobic endurance using an arm ergometer has been prescribed starting with low load for 1-minute bouts and progressing to 20 minutes at loads of up to 25 watts.[3] Walking, jogging, bicycling, and swimming at moderate intensities (60% to 75% of maximum heart rate) have also been used as adjuncts to resistance exercises. Clients should be reassessed weekly for positive or negative effects on limb volume measurements and for their tolerance to the prescribed exercise program. Clients should be encouraged to maintain a regular exercise program for their cardiovascular health and to sustain the recovery of lymphatic functions in their affected limb.

References

1. Hayes SC, Reul-Hirche H, Turner J. Exercise and secondary lymphedema: Safety, potential benefits, and research issues. Med Sci Sports Exerc 41(3):483-489, 2009.
2. Sagen A, Kåresen R, Risberg MA. Physical activity for the affected limb and arm lymphedema after breast cancer surgery: A prospective, randomized controlled trial with two years follow-up. Acta Oncol Jun 23:1-9, 2009.
3. McKenzie DC, Kalda AL. Effect of upper extremity exercise on secondary lymphedema in breast cancer patients: A pilot study. J Clin Oncol 21(3):463-466, 2003.
4. Ahmed RL, Thomas W, Yee D, et al. Randomized controlled trial of weight training and lymphedema in breast cancer survivors. J Clin Oncol 24(18):2765-2772, 2006.
5. Bicego D, Brown K, Ruddick M, et al. Exercise for women with or at risk for breast cancer-related lymphedema. Phys Ther 86(10):1398-1405, 2006.
6. Schmitz KH, Ahmed RL, Troxel A, et al. Weight-lifting in women with breast-cancer–related lymphedema. N Engl J Med 361(7):664-673, 2009.
7. Johansson K, Tibe K, Weibull A, et al. Low-intensity resistance exercise for breast cancer patients with arm lymphedema with or without compression sleeve. Lymphology 38(4):167-180, 2005.

METABOLIC SYNDROME

Overview of Metabolic Syndrome

Metabolic syndrome is a collection of factors associated with central obesity. Central obesity is indicated by waist circumferences of ≥94 cm for men and >80 cm for women. Metabolic syndrome is further determined by any two of the following: raised triglycerides, reduced high-density lipoprotein cholesterol, raised blood pressure, and raised fasting plasma glucose levels or type 2 diabetes.[1,2] Clinical management of this syndrome is focused on controlling its risk factors, especially atherosclerosis. Clients with metabolic syndrome have impaired endurance, primarily related to a sedentary lifestyle. Endurance impairments are exacerbated by the development of cardiovascular disease and complications related to type 2 diabetes. Clients using medications for prevention and treatment of cardiovascular disease or type 2 diabetes will need regular evaluation for the effectiveness of these medications.

Clinical Management Goals for Management of Metabolic Syndrome

Prevent cardiovascular disease
Increase physical activities
Reduce low-density lipoprotein
  cholesterol levels

Prevention/treatment of type 2 diabetes
Reduce intake of saturated fats and cholesterol
Reduce elevated blood pressure levels

Comorbidities to Consider

• Clients with metabolic syndrome have a higher risk for cardiovascular disease and type 2 diabetes.

Client Examination

Keys to Examination of Clients

• Clients need regular examinations to assess blood pressure, fasting blood glucose level, and lipid levels.
• Discuss with these clients their previous experiences, beliefs, and other conditions that will make them reluctant to begin an exercise program.

Recommended Baseline Testing of Fitness Levels

• Assess endurance with a half-mile walk, 6-minute walk, or 10-meter walk, depending on the client's functional status.[3]
• Determine body mass index and waist circumference to assess body composition.[3]
• Client's heart rate, blood pressure, and perceived exertion levels should be regularly assessed at beginning of exercise program.

Exercise Prescription

Type: Walking, aquatic exercise, weight training
Intensity: 40%–70% of maximum capacity[3,4]
Duration: Start at 15–20 minutes, progress to 60 minutes
Frequency: 5–7 days per week

Getting Started

Walking is the easiest form of exercise to begin and maintain. Clients may benefit from using a pedometer to assess their daily activity levels and to encourage them to walk throughout the day to increase their caloric output. Multiple forms of aerobic exercise are recommended for these clients to improve adherence and to avoid overuse conditions. Clients with morbid obesity may best start an exercise program using aquatic activities. Resistive exercise training is also recommended for these clients, as it improves insulin sensitivity and may enhance metabolism of adipose tissue in the abdominal region.[5] A goal of 150 to 250 minutes of total physical activity per week or 1500 to 1800 kcal of physical activities along with appropriate caloric intake limits will bring about weight loss.[6] Provide ongoing counseling on the benefits of an exercise program, and allow these clients to help design their exercise program. Clients should progress the duration and frequency of their exercise program to promote weight loss and decrease waist circumference to levels that will reduce their risk for cardiovascular and metabolic diseases. Clients should be encouraged to maintain a regular exercise program for a minimum of 5 days per week for 30 minutes to maintain weight loss.

References

1. Alberti KG, Zimmet P, Shaw J. The metabolic syndrome, a new worldwide definition. Lancet 366: 1059-1062, 2005.
2. American Heart Association—Metabolic Syndrome. http://www.americanheart.org/presenter.jhtml?identifier=4756. Accessed July 3, 2009.
3. Humphrey R, Tepper SH. Prevention and wellness: Practical strategies in clinical practice to management diabetic risk and metabolic syndrome. PT 2009: Annual Conference and Exposition, Baltimore.
4. ACSM Guidelines for Exercise Testing and Prescription, 7th ed Baltimore, Williams & Wilkins: 2005.
5. Tresierras MA, Balady GJ. Resistance training in the treatment of diabetes and obesity: Mechanisms and outcomes. J Cardiopul Rehabil Prev 29(2):67-75, 2009.
6. Donnelly JE, Blair SN, Jakicic JM, et al. American College of Sports Medicine position stand: Appropriate physical activity intervention strategies for weight loss and prevention of weight regain for adults. Med Sci Sports Exerc 41(2):459-471, 2009.

MULTIPLE SCLEROSIS (MS)

Overview of MS

MS is characterized by the development of sclerotic plaques in the central nervous system, which results in blocked or slowed neural transmissions. MS has episodes of increased symptoms followed by periods of recovery. There are four subtypes, based on the pattern of progression of the disease. Initial symptoms are sensory changes, visual deficits, muscle weakness, and balance impairments. Diagnosis of MS is based on the clinical presentation of symptoms and the identification of lesions on magnetic resonance imaging (MRI) of the central nervous system. Clients with MS have periods of increased fatigue and weakness, resulting in limited daily activities. Inactivity is linked to decreased aerobic capacity, reduced muscle strength, increased fatigue, and reduced maximum gait velocity.[1]

Comorbidities to Consider

- Progression of the disease process results in sensory deficits, with poor coordination and balance with movements.

Client Examination

Keys to Examination of Clients

- MRI of the central nervous system will identify the location and extent of sclerotic plaques, which may assist in understanding the extent and progression of the disease.
- Determine fatigue levels before starting exercise and as an ongoing assessment for prescribing exercise intensities and durations.
- Determine the progression of the disease and the prognosis for improvement in function with the Kurtzke Expanded Disability Status Scale.[2]

Recommended Baseline Testing of Fitness Levels

- A 10-meter and a 6-minute walk have been used to assess mobility and endurance in clients.[1]
- Isometric tests of muscle strength and functional assessments can be used to determine a baseline of strength measurements.[3,4] Clients' overall mobility and activities should be assessed to determine the quality and amount of their movement.

Exercise Prescription

Type: Walking, cycle ergometry, and aquatic exercise
Intensity: Start at 50%–70% of V_{O_2} maximum or 60%–80% of maximum heart rate[1]
Duration: 10–20 minutes
Frequency: Two to three sessions per week

Getting Started

A combination of endurance and resistive training is recommended. Endurance training is appropriate for clients with minimal to moderate disability levels.[1,5] Clients with no disability can participate in road running, bicycling, and recreational activities. The exercise environment must be controlled as many clients experience heat intolerance. Training should be increased in duration and frequency according to baseline testing and the client's control of fatigue level.

Resistive training, especially for the lower extremities, using weight training equipment is recommended for starting an exercise program.[1] A circuit of five to eight upper and lower extremity resistive exercises at an intensity allowing for 15 repetitions for one to three sets is recommended.[1,4] The emphasis should be on lower extremity exercises as these muscle groups are commonly affected the disease, and improvements in strength are associated with improvements in activities. The exercises can be performed two to three times per week and can be used in combination with endurance activities.

References

1. Dalgas U, Ingemann-Hansen T, Stenager E. Physical exercise and MS recommendations. Int Multiple Sclerosis J 16(1):5-11, 2009.
2. Kurtzke JF. Historical and clinical perspectives of the expanded disability status scale. Neuroepidemiology 31(1):1-9, 2008.
3. Dalgas U, Stenager E, Jakobsen J, et al. Resistance training improves muscle strength and functional capacity in multiple sclerosis. Neurology 73(18):1478-1484, 2009.
4. Dalgas U, Stenager E, Ingemann-Hansen T. Multiple sclerosis and physical exercise: Recommendations for the application of resistance, endurance, and combined training. Multiple Sclerosis 2008;14(1):35-53.
5. Rietberg MB, Brooks D, Uitdehaag BM, et al. Exercise therapy for multiple sclerosis. Cochrane Database Syst Rev Jan 25;(1):CD003980, 2005.

OBESITY

Overview of Obesity

Obesity is due to a combination of genetic, environmental, and behavioral factors that results in an energy imbalance to promote excessive fat storage.[1] Obesity can be defined by a client's body weight, body fat percentages, and body mass index (BMI). The World Health Organization uses a BMI of >30 as the cutoff for class 1 obesity, with levels of >35 for class 2 and >40 for class 3.[2] Waist circumference can be used with BMI to assess health risks related to obesity. Circumferences of ≥88 cm for women and ≥102 cm for men indicate greater risk for disease. Sedentary lifestyle is a significant risk factor for obesity and the primary cause of endurance impairments for individuals with obesity.[3] Clients need regular examinations to assess blood pressure, blood glucose, and lipid levels. Clients benefit from interdisciplinary management that may include pharmacologic agents, nutritional counseling, and behavioral therapy.[1]

Comorbidities to Consider

- Obesity is a significant risk factor for developing diabetes, heart disease, and a number of other medical conditions.[3]

Obesity Is an Increased Risk for:

Type 2 diabetes	Hirsutism
Heart disease	Depression
Stroke	Stress incontinence
Osteoarthritis	Pregnancy complications
Asthma	Surgical complications
Cancer	Incontinence
Gallbladder disease	Sleep apnea

Client Examination

Keys to Examination of Clients

- Take considerable time to talk with your clients with obesity to understand their previous experiences and beliefs about exercise before developing a plan. These individuals should be counseled on the benefits of an exercise program and must be allowed to help design their exercise program.
- A medical history will help identify conditions that may limit their exercise tolerance.
- Exercise activities may exacerbate existing degenerative conditions, cause chafing and skin disorders, and may make an individual susceptible to falling and heat intolerance.
- Assess client's body composition, BMI, and waist circumference before the client begins an exercise program.

Recommended Baseline Testing of Fitness Levels

- Based on the client's current functional status, determine a method for assessing the individual's exercise tolerance. The most common methods for clients with obesity are the half-mile walk, 6-minute walk, or the 10-meter walk.[4,5]
- The client's heart rate, blood pressure, and perceived exertion levels should be regularly assessed at the outset of the exercise program.

Exercise Prescription

Type: Walking, aquatic exercise, weight training
Intensity: Low to moderate intensities, 40%–70% of maximum VO_2 -
Duration: Up to 60 minutes
Frequency: Five to seven times per week.

Getting Started

Group exercise can be recommended for those clients with similar weight-loss challenges. Clients with morbid obesity may best start an exercise program using aquatic activities.[3] Recommend that clients maintain a low level of intensity for walking and other aerobic activities while they increase the duration and frequency of their exercise program.[5] Consider the use of strength training as an adjunct to aerobic forms of exercise, as such training has been used to maintain resting metabolic rates in men undergoing weight loss.[3] Clients may benefit from using a pedometer to assess their daily activity levels and to encourage them to use walking throughout the day to increase their caloric output. Clients using a pedometer should be using at least 5000 steps per day, with a goal of increasing daily walking up to 10,000 steps. Clients may choose a number of methods for assessing their physical activity level and setting appropriate goals for weight loss. The Compendium of Physical Activities can be used to identify daily activities used to increase daily caloric output.[6] A goal of 150 to 250 minutes of physical activity per week, or 1500 to 1800 kcal of physical activity along with appropriate caloric intake limits, will bring about weight loss.[7,8] Clients should try different modes of exercise to encourage them to maintain their exercise program. Clients should be encouraged to maintain a regular exercise program for a minimum of 5 days per peak to maintain weight loss, but no evidence is available to indicate the most appropriate level of weekly exercise needed to maintain weight loss.[8]

References

1. Racette SB, Deusinger SS, Deusinger RH. Obesity: Overview of prevalence, etiology, and treatment. Phys Ther 83:276-287, 2003.
2. World Health Organization BMI classification. http://apps.who.int/bmi/index.jsp?introPage=intro_3.html. Accessed November 24, 2009.
3. Surgeon general's call to action to prevent and decrease overweight and obesity. http://www.surgeongeneral.gov/topics/obesity/calltoaction/toc.htm. Accessed November 24, 2009.
4. ACSM Guidelines for Exercise Testing and Prescription, 7th ed. Baltimore: Williams & Wilkins, 2005.
5. Humphrey R, Tepper SH. Prevention and wellness: Practical strategies in clinical practice to management of diabetic risk and metabolic syndrome. PT 2009: Annual Conference and Exposition, Baltimore.

6. Compendium of physical activities tracking guide. http://prevention.sph.sc.edu/tools/docs/documents_compendium.pdf. Accessed November 24, 2009.
7. Stiegler P, Cunliffe A. The role of diet and exercise for the maintenance of fat-free mass and resting metabolic rate during weight loss. Sports Med 36(3):239-262, 2006.
8. Donnelly JE, Blair SN, Jakicic JM, et al. American College of Sports Medicine position stand. Appropriate physical activity intervention strategies for weight loss and prevention of weight regain for adults. Med Sci Sports Exerc 41(2):459-471, 2009.

ORGAN TRANSPLANTATION, KIDNEY AND LIVER

Overview of Kidney and Liver Organ Transplantation

Kidneys and livers comprise the greatest number of successful transplantations. The majority of candidates for kidney transplants have end-stage kidney disease resulting from type 1 diabetes, and the majority of liver transplants are for individuals with end-stage liver disease. The number of successful candidates for these transplants has increased due to an increased understanding controlling organ rejection and other complications of these disease processes. Transplant rejection occurs in 10% to 20% of all cases, usually within the first 3 months, but rejection can occur years later. Post-transplant musculoskeletal pain, especially the knee and ankle joints, is common in the first 6 months, affecting up to 35% of individuals receiving a renal transplant and 25% of liver transplants. After receiving a kidney or liver, clients may have limited mobility and endurance from excessive fatigue. Complications from their diseases and side effects of their numerous drugs affect physical activity.

Comorbidities to Consider

- Clients may have significant cardiopulmonary and musculoskeletal complications after organ transplantation. Recipients of kidneys are at increased risk of osteoporosis, osteonecrosis, sensory polyneuropathy, and the fractures associated with these conditions.[1] Excessive body fat mass has been associated with physical inactivity and steroid use in clients after transplantation.[2,3]

Client Examination

Keys to Examination of Clients

- Assess the results of recent tests for blood counts and for cardiac and pulmonary function.
- Measure fatigue levels before and during exercise programs.[3,4]
- Employ the Health-Related Quality of Life inventory to assess clients' current physical function, pain, and general health status.[5]

Recommended Baseline Testing of Fitness Levels

- Aerobic capacity can be assessed by walking or treadmill tests to determine peak aerobic capacity and maximum heart rate.
- Strength of the large muscle group has been assessed by isometric or isokinetic testing.
- Screen for limited mobility and signs of degenerative conditions to prescribe the appropriate types and parameters of exercise.

Exercise Prescription

Type: Walking, cycling, and home-based activities[2,6]
Intensity: Start at 60%–65% of maximum heart rate
Duration: Progress to 30 minutes
Frequency: Three times per week

Getting Started

A fitness support group may benefit clients having similar procedures and disease processes.[7] Circuit resistance training is recommended for clients with a stable health status, beginning with low intensities with 12 to 15 repetitions for one to two sets of upper and lower extremity exercises. Such exercises can be used to improve muscle strength and functional levels. Aerobic and resistive training programs can be alternated on a daily basis to maintain a regular behavior of exercise while allowing for recovery from each exercise session. By engaging in unfamiliar exercise activities, clients may fear injuring their joints and transplanted organ.[8] Aerobic activities can be progressed to 75% to 80% of maximum heart rate for 45 to 60 minutes three to five times per week. Clients who reach a stable level of health can return to recreational activities; some clients may choose to participate in Transplant Games.[9]

References

1. Gevirtz C. Post-transplantation pain syndromes. Topics Pain Manage 23(8):1-6, 2008.
2. Krasnoff JB, Vintro AQ, Ascher NL, et al. A randomized trial of exercise and dietary counseling after liver transplantation. Am J Transplant 6(8):1896-1905, 2006.
3. Macdonald JH, Kirkman D, Jibani M. Kidney transplantation: A systematic review of interventional and observational studies of physical activity on intermediate outcomes. Adv Chronic Kidney Dis 16(6): 482-500, 2009.
4. van Ginneken BT, van den Berg-Emons RJ, van der Windt A, et al. Persistent fatigue in liver transplant recipients: A two-year follow-up study. Clin Transplant Sep 11, 2009.
5. Health-related quality of life. http://www.cdc.gov/hrqol/hrqol14_measure.htm. Accessed February 9, 2010.
6. Gordon EJ, Prohaska T, Siminoff LA, et al. Needed: Tailored exercise regimens for kidney transplant recipients. Am J Kidney Dis 45(4):769-774, 2005.
7. Gentry AC, Belza B, Simpson T. Fitness support group for organ transplant recipients: Self-management, self-efficacy and health status. J Adv Nurs 65(11):2419-2425, 2009.
8. Sánchez ZV, Cashion AK, Cowan PA, et al. Perceived barriers and facilitators to physical activity in kidney transplant recipients. Prog Transplant 17(4):324-331, 2007.
9. World Transplant Games Federation. http://www.wtgf.org/. Accessed November 5, 2009.

OSTEOARTHRITIS

Overview of Osteoarthritis

Osteoarthritis refers to a group of conditions characterized by progressive degeneration of articular cartilage, subchondral bone, and other joint structures. The disease process usually begins with excessive or abnormal mechanical stresses to the articular surfaces, with a chronic inflammatory process leading to the characteristic changes of all the joint structures. Radiographic appearance of osteoarthritis is characterized by loss of joint space, subchondral bone sclerosis, and osteophyte formations. Radiographic signs for the extent of joint changes may not correlate strongly with the client's current symptoms. Weight-bearing joints of the lower extremities and the spine are affected most often. Clients with this condition experience significant joint pain and stiffness that limit mobility and result in diminished daily activities.[1] As the condition progresses, the client experiences more fatigue and discomfort with daily activities and may choose to self-limit activities to reduce these symptoms. Exercise programs have been found to be highly effective for the treatment of osteoarthritis.[2]

Effects of Exercise Programs on Clients With Osteoarthritis

Pain reduction   Improved physical function
Weight reduction   Decreased self-reported disability levels

Comorbidities to Consider

- Reduced physical activities typically lead to weight gain and a progression of atherosclerosis that can exacerbate the client endurance impairment and further reduce tolerance to activities.[3]

Client Examination

Keys to Examination of Clients

- Examine images or imaging reports to assess the extent of osteoarthritic changes to joint structures.
- Employ the Western Ontario and McMaster Osteoarthritis Index (WOMAC) to assess the client's pain, disability, and joint stiffness.[4]
- Discuss with clients their social support, understanding of their disease process, and self-efficacy for maintaining an exercise program.[5,6]

Recommended Baseline Testing of Fitness Levels

- Walking tests can be performed to assess a client's walking velocity and tolerance to endurance activities.[3,7] Exercise capacity assessed with cycling may be preferred by clients with significant lower extremity osteoarthritis.
- Use functional activities of squatting or stepping as well as strength assessments for lower extremity muscle groups.[5,7]

Exercise Prescription

Type: Walking, cycling, aquatic activities, weight training
Intensity: Start at low intensities
Duration: Start at 10–20 minutes
Frequency: Three to five times per week

Getting Started

Aerobic activities are recommended for clients with osteoarthritis for promoting weight loss and improving physical function.[2,8] Clients beginning an exercise program should be allowed to self-select the intensity of their exercise, as joint pain will be a limiting factor.[7,8] Clients should be encouraged to increase their intensity to a level of 60% to 80% of their maximum heart rate for weight loss and cardiovascular benefits. Aquatic exercise has been recommended, but most of the benefits have been shown to be short-term and mostly to those new to exercising.[9] Tai chi has been used for pain control but has not been found to improve physical function.[10] Resistance exercise, with light to moderate intensity for lower-extremity muscle groups, especially the knee extensors and flexors, is recommended.[5]

Clients should be educated on how to avoid excessive joint stresses by alternating types of activities, avoiding long-term weight-bearing positions and performing exercises with appropriate postures and movements. Clients can progress to an independent program to maintain their fitness level and physical function. Clients may benefit from periodic re-evaluation of their physical function and exercise program to promote adherence to the program. Clients may also benefit from a consultation with a dietitian to assist in a weight loss program, if indicated.

References

1. Deyle GD, Allison SC, Matekel RL, et al. Physical therapy treatment effectiveness for osteoarthritis of the knee: A randomized comparison of supervised clinical exercise and manual therapy procedures versus a home exercise program. Phys Ther 85(12):1301-1317, 2005.
2. Jamtvedt G, Dahm KT, Christie A, et al. Physical therapy interventions for patients with osteoarthritis of the knee: An overview of systematic reviews. Phys Ther 88(1):123-136, 2008.
3. Messier SP. Obesity and osteoarthritis: Disease genesis and nonpharmacologic weight management. Rheum Dis Clin North Am 34(3):713-729, 2008.
4. WOMAC Osteoarthritis Index. http://www.womac.org/womac/. Accessed October 17, 2009.
5. Lange AK, Vanwanseele B, Fiatarone Singh MA. Strength training for treatment of osteoarthritis of the knee: A systematic review. Arthritis Rheum 59(10):1488-1494, 2008.
6. Marks R, Allegrante JP. Chronic osteoarthritis and adherence to exercise: A review of the literature. J Aging Phys Act. 13(4):434-460, 2005.
7. Bruno M, Cummins S, Gaudiano L, et al. Effectiveness of two Arthritis Foundation programs: Walk With Ease, and YOU Can Break the Pain Cycle. Clin Interv Aging 1(3):295-306, 2006.
8. Roddy E, Zhang W, Doherty M, et al. Evidence-based recommendations for the role of exercise in the management of osteoarthritis of the hip or knee: The MOVE consensus. Rheumatol (Oxford) 44(1):67-73, 2005.
9. Bartels EM, Lund H, Hagen KB, et al. Aquatic exercise for the treatment of knee and hip osteoarthritis. Cochrane Database Syst Rev Oct 17;(4):CD005523, 2007.
10. Lee MS, Pittler MH, Ernst E. Tai chi for osteoarthritis: A systematic review. Clin Rheumatol 27(2): 211-218, 2008.

OSTEOMYELITIS

Overview of Osteomyelitis

This condition is an inflammation of bony tissues secondary to an infection. Chronic osteomyelitis can lead to surgical removal of connective tissues and amputations. Chronic infections and surgical procedures can also lead to limited joint and tissue mobility. The tibia and femur are most susceptible to osteomyelitis after a traumatic injury. Clients will benefit from the potential effects of exercise to enhance their immune system and to mediate the effects of stress and depression. Clients will have limited activities due to the effects of the infections and complications, leading to deconditioning.[1] Inflammation of bony tissues is painful and limits the client's ability to initiate movement.

Comorbidities to Consider

- Conditions that may compromise the immune system in these clients include diabetes mellitus, spinal cord injury, alcoholism, and malnutrition.

Client Examination

Keys to Examination of Clients

- Review reports of laboratory tests and cultures taken of infected tissues to determine the type and extent of the infection.
- Radiographs and computed tomography scans of the affected area can provide information about the extent of bony tissue damage.
- Patients with limited mobility can be assessed for their level of independence with transfers and ambulation.

Recommended Baseline Testing of Fitness Levels

- Assessments of endurance, strength, and mobility need to be designed to meet the current abilities of the client.[2]
- Clients unable to ambulate can use an upper body ergometer or an endurance test using a wheelchair to provide information about their exercise tolerance.[3]

Exercise Prescription

Type: Cycling, arm ergometry, weight training
Intensity: Low to moderate intensities
Duration: 10–20 minutes
Frequency: Three to five times per week

Getting Started

Treatment programs for osteomyelitis can become complex and will require ongoing monitoring of vital signs, pain from the affected area, and assessments of wound healing. Prevention of movement dysfunctions will require ongoing monitoring of movement, strength, and weight-bearing tolerance. Clients with limited lower extremity weight bearing can perform arm ergometry or use a wheelchair.[1] Repetitive movements using hand weights or pulleys allow for a variety of movements with concentric and eccentric muscle contractions. Clients with infectious processes may not be able to move the extremity due to discomfort. Aseptic techniques are very important when treating a client with a history of osteomyelitis.

Clients benefit from endurance activities progressed to 40% to 65% of predicted maximum heart rate for 30 to 40 minutes. Clients using an arm ergometer can use ratings of perceived exertion to control their exercise intentsity.[4] Intense exercise activities need to be avoided for these clients as these may produce muscle soreness and may affect the immune system negatively. Resistive exercises should also use low to moderate intensities with sets of 10 to 20 repetitions. Clients will need ongoing assessment and adjustment to their rehabilitation and exercise programs. Clients should understand how their exercise program contributes to their overall health and abilities to perform their regular activities. Clients who have undergone lower-extremity amputation benefit from an exercise program to improve their endurance in preparation for prosthetic training.

References

1. Pedersen BK, Hoffman-Goetz L. Exercise and the immune system: Regulation, integration, and adaptation. Physiol Rev 80:1055-1081, 2000.
2. Johnston B, Conly J. Osteomyelitis management: More art than science? Can J Infect Dis Med Microbiol 18(2):115-118, 2007.
3. Ilias NA, Xian H, Inman C, et al. Arm exercise testing predicts clinical outcome. Am Heart J 157(1):69-76, 2009.
4. Kang J, Chaloupka EC, Mastrangelo MA, et al. Regulating exercise intensity using ratings of perceived exertion during arm and leg ergometry. Eur J Appl Physiol Occup Physiol 78(3):241-246, 1998.

OSTEOPOROSIS

Overview of Osteoporosis

Osteoporosis is the loss of bone tissue leading to decreased bone density. Poor acquisition of bone density in youth and accelerated bone density loss during aging are the primary reasons for developing osteoporosis. Bone density acquisition and loss are regulated by genetic and environmental factors. Primary osteoporosis is due to loss of estrogen and aging, whereas secondary osteoporosis is due to conditions or medications that accelerate bone loss. Risk factors for developing osteoporosis are genetic, behavioral, and nutritional.[1] Bone mineral density (BMD) is assessed by passing low-level radiation through the bone to estimate the level of bone mineral content. Tests are typically taken of the vertebral spine, neck of the femur, and wrist bones. Individuals with a BMD T-score of -2.5 or less are diagnosed with osteoporosis. Individuals with primary osteoporosis do not have specific causes for endurance impairments, outside of their normal limitations based on age and activity level. Those with secondary osteoporosis may have endurance impairments associated with another chronic condition. Management of osteoporosis requires the combination of factors to control the loss of bone density.[2]

Recommended Treatments for Clients With Osteoporosis

Adequate intake of calcium and vitamin D

Avoidance of tobacco

Pharmacologic therapies

Regular weight-bearing exercise

Avoidance of excessive alcohol intake

Falls prevention

Comorbidities to Consider

- Postural changes and vertebral compression fractures are common complications associated with osteoporosis.

Client Examination

Keys to the Examination of the Client

- Assess the risk of fracture using the World Health Organization's Fracture Risk Assessment Tool (FRAX).[3]
- Because of the increased risk of fracture due to falling, assessment of balance and ongoing prevention of falling will be needed during exercise sessions.
- A BMD test after 6 months of exercise may help determine the benefit of a specific exercise program.

Recommended Baseline Testing of Fitness Levels

- Determine an aerobic capacity and strength assessment based on the client's functional status and plans for starting an exercise program.

Exercise Prescription

Type: Weight-bearing activities and weight training
Intensity: Moderate intensities
Duration: Start at 20–30 minutes
Frequency: Three to five times per week

Getting Started

Aerobic activities of walking, jogging, or dancing combined with a strength training program are recommended for patients with osteoporosis. There are no absolute restrictions for clients with primary osteoporosis; however, individuals with secondary osteoporosis may have limited ability to exercise due to other chronic conditions Exercise prescriptions are directed at slowing the rate of loss of bone density as there is limited evidence for the effects of exercise to reverse the pathogenesis associated with osteoporosis.[4]

Aerobic exercises should emphasize the overall weekly volume (sessions and time per session) of activities. Strength training should be performed with a high intensity using the resistance equal to 80% of a one-repetition maximum. Exercises can be performed with two to three sets of 8 to 10 repetitions.[1] Handheld weights are preferred as they allow for the most options for standing exercises with weight bearing through the extremities and trunk.[1,4] A client without previous exercise experience can slowly increase the session time and time per session over 8 weeks. Strength-training sessions can be progressed by adding different types of exercises, preferably those that allow the client to stand or sit while exercising. Balance training and fall prevention education have also been included in these programs to decrease risk of falls that result in fractures.[1,4] Recent studies suggest exercising on a low-frequency vibratory platform may enhance the effects for BMD.[5]

References

1. Downey PA, Siegel MI. Bone biology and the clinical implications for osteoporosis. Phys Ther 86:77-91, 2006.
2. National Osteoporosis Foundation. http://www.nof.org/professionals/pdfs/NOF_ClinicianGuide2009_v7.pdf. Accessed March 10, 2010.
3. Fracture Risk Assessment. www.shef.ac.uk/FRAX/. Accessed November 25, 2009.
4. Pedersen BK, Saltin B. Evidence for prescribing exercise as therapy in chronic disease. Scand J Med Sci Sports 16(Suppl 1):3-63, 2006.
5. Gusi N, Raimundo A, Leal A. Low-frequency vibratory exercise reduces the risk of bone fracture more than walking: A randomized controlled trial. BMC Musculoskeletal Disord 30(7):92, 2006.

PARKINSON'S DISEASE

Overview of Parkinson's Disease

This is a chronic progressive disease involving the subcortical gray matter of the basal ganglia. Most cases are due to a genetic defect, with toxic and infectious exposures being risk factors. The disease progresses as the substantia nigra of the basal ganglia loses its ability to produce dopamine.[1] Because the basal ganglia is important for the initiation and control of motor behaviors, the progression of the disease significantly alters how movements occur, resulting in slowing of movement and loss of coordination. A decrease in daily activities and social participation results in deconditioning and a decrease in cardiovascular functions. The Unified Parkinson's Disease Rating Scale and the Hoehn and Yahr Classification of Disability are used to determine disease progression.[1]

Hoehn and Yahr Classification of Disability

Stage 1: Minimal disability, unilateral involvement
Stage 2: Minimal bilateral involvement, balance not impaired
Stage 3: Impaired righting reflexes, unsteadiness but lives independently
Stage 4: Severe symptoms, standing and walking possible with assistance
Stage 5: Confined to bed or wheelchair

Comorbidities to Consider

- Clients may develop depression and dementia that limit activities, and they may have dyspnea, rapid heart rate, and sweating with physical activities.

Client Examination

Keys to Examination of Clients

- This condition is diagnosed based on the presentation of tremor, rigidity, bradykinesia, and akinesia. The concentration of dopamine transporters can be measured through computed tomography scans.
- Screen the client's ability to move in a safe manner and for risk of falling with sitting and standing activities.

Recommended Baseline Testing of Fitness Levels

- Aerobic fitness can be assessed with the 2- or 6-minute walk tests.[2]
- Assess for strength, mobility, and balance based on the client's status and disease progression.

Exercise Prescription

Type: Walking, treadmill walking, stationary bicyling[3,4]
Intensity: Low to moderate intensities
Duration: 20–30 minutes
Frequency: Four times per week

Getting Started

Aerobic exercises performed for 6 weeks have resulted in significant changes in gait and quality of life measures and improved the efficacy of the medication levodopa.[5,6] The intensity of the exercise should be prescribed for each client, with a goal of exercising at 60% to 80% of maximum heart rate. Balance and sensorimotor agility activities can be incorporated into a client's daily activities and recreational pursuits.[7] Exercise and therapies that provide for sensorimotor agility, such as tai chi, kayaking, and Pilates, have also been advocated for these clients.[7,8] Clients may need to time the use of their medications to diminish their rigidity, tremor, and akinesia during exercise sessions. The regulation of medications for Parkinson's and its side effects can be a significant barrier to regular exercise participation. Clients should be encouraged to maintain or increase their level of independent exercise, depending on the progressions of symptoms and their preference for engaging in aerobic and recreational activities.

References

1. National Parkinson Foundation. http://www.parkinson.org/Page.aspx?&pid=367&srcid=230. Accessed November 24, 2009.
2. White DK, Wagenaar RC, Ellis TD, et al. Changes in walking activity and endurance following rehabilitation for people with Parkinson disease. Arch Phys Med Rehabil 90(1):43-50, 2009.
3. Crizzle AM, Newhouse IJ. Is physical exercise beneficial for persons with Parkinson's disease? Clin J Sport Med 16(5):422-425, 2006.
4. Goodwin VA, Richards SH, Taylor RS, et al. The effectiveness of exercise interventions for people with Parkinson's disease: A systematic review and meta-analysis. Movement Disord 23(5):631-640, 2008.
5. Herman T, Giladi N, Gruendlinger L, et al. Six weeks of intensive treadmill training improves gait and quality of life in patients with Parkinson's disease: A pilot study. Arch Phys Med Rehabil 88(9): 1154-1158, 2007.
6. Muhlack S, Welnic J, Woitalla D, et al. Exercise improves efficacy of levodopa in patients with Parkinson's disease. Movement Disord 22(3):427-430, 2007.
7. Kwakkel G, de Goede CJ, van Wegen EE. Impact of physical therapy for Parkinson's disease: A critical review of the literature. Parkinsonism Related Disord 13(Suppl 3):S478-487, 2007.
8. King LA, Horak FB. Delaying mobility disability in people with Parkinson disease using a sensorimotor agility exercise program. Phys Ther 89(4):384-393, 2009.

PERIPHERAL ARTERIAL DISEASE (PAD)

Overview of PAD

PAD results from atherosclerosis of the arteries that extend through the extremities. Narrowing of the arteries reduces blood flow to the limbs, which results in pain, pallor, and paresthesias. Intermittent claudication is associated with PAD, with individuals describing burning and cramping pain in the legs during walking activities. Risk factors for PAD include smoking, hypertension, and low levels of high-density lipoprotein cholesterol. Clients with PAD have limited standing and walking abilities due to intermittent claudication, which slows their walking speed and changes their gait pattern. The presence of coronary heart disease also limits their capacity for physical activities. As the disease process advances, the patient tolerates fewer standing and walking activities.

Common Signs and Symptoms of Arterial Insufficiency

Painful walking	Redness in the distal limb
Elevated lower extremity develops pallor	Poor venous filling after extremity is elevated
Skin dryness	Tissue necrosis

Comorbidities to Consider

• Individuals with PAD typically also have coronary heart and cardiovascular disease.

Client Examination

Keys to Examination of Clients

• Assess for signs of hypertension and other signs of cardiovascular disease.
• Pulses and skin color and intactness at the feet and ankles should be assessed.
• Determine an ankle-brachial index by taking systolic blood pressure at the ankle and the arm. Ratios of ankle-to-arm pressure below 0.90 indicate a significant decrease in systolic pressures in the lower extremities.

Recommended Baseline Testing of Fitness Levels

• A walking or treadmill walking test is used to determine a baseline for distances. The client is asked to walk at a normal pace until unable to walk due to leg pain. The walking distance before the initiation of leg symptoms and absolute walking distance are noted for baseline measurement.[1]

Exercise Prescription

Type: Walking, treadmill walking, and lower-extremity exercises
Intensity: Mild to moderate intensities
Duration: 3–5-minute bouts with rest periods
Frequency: Three to five times per week

Getting Started

Walking on a treadmill is the most effective mode of exercise to control intensity and duration of walking. Clients may need to use an assistive device or the railing of the treadmill to initiate the program. Clients with severe leg pain or pain at rest may need to start their exercise program using a cycle ergometer. Because clients with PAD typically have severe pain with walking activities, the purpose of testing and exercising should be thoroughly discussed before starting the program. Clients with PAD may experience unsteadiness and balance problems as the complaints of intermittent claudication increase; clients may self-limit their activities to avoid or in expectation of leg pain. Walking programs of mild to moderate intensity have been shown to be successful for increasing pain-free walking distances by improving lower extremity circulation and walking economy.[2-4] Recommended walking programs include setting the speed of the treadmill so that the client has moderate claudication symptoms within 3 to 5 minutes, allowing the client to take a sitting rest until the symptoms subside and then return to treadmill at the same speed. The initial goal is to complete a total of 30 minutes of walking, increasing to 50 minutes of walking. Adjust the intensity when the client can walk 8 to 10 minutes before experiencing moderate symptoms.[4] Other programs set the walking speed at 2 m.p.h. and gradually increase the grade of the treadmill to increase walking intensity.[3] Walking programs should be performed three to five times per week for at least 12 weeks to significantly improve the client's daily activity level. Supervised exercise programs, because they involve the provocation of claudication symptoms, have been shown to be more successful than independent exercise programs.[1,4,5] Resistance training program have used intensities increasing from 50% to 80% of a one-repetition using three sets of eight repetitions.[5] Clients with PAD should be counseled to continue with an exercise program to maintain the effects for their intermittent claudication, as well as manage their coronary heart disease.

References

1. Wind J, Koelemay MJ. Exercise therapy and the additional effect of supervision of exercise therapy in patients with intermittent claudication: Systematic review of randomized controlled trials. Eur J Vasc Endovasc Surg 34(1):1-9, 2007.
2. Gardner AW, Katzel LI, Sorkin JD, et al. Exercise rehabilitation improves functional outcomes and peripheral circulation in patient with intermittent claudication: A randomized controlled trial. J Am Geriatr Soc 49(6):755-762, 2001.
3. Falcone RA, Hirsch AT, Regensteiner JG, et al. Peripheral arterial disease rehabilitation: A review. J Cardiopulmonary Rehabil 23(3):170-175, 2003.
4. Hirsch AT, Haskal ZJ, Hertzer NR. ACC/AHA 2005 guidelines for the management of patients with peripheral arterial disease. Circulation 21;113(11):463-654, 2006.
5. McDermott MM, Ades P, Guralnik JM, et al. Treadmill exercise and resistance training in patients with peripheral arterial disease with and without intermittent claudication: A randomized controlled trial. JAMA 301(2):165-174, 2009.

POST-POLIO SYNDROME

Overview of Post-Polio Syndrome

This condition is a slowly progressive disorder consisting of muscular atrophy, pain, and fatigue that occurs decades after an acute polio paralytic episode. This syndrome results when the motor neurons that provided re-innervation of muscle fibers begin to prune back their axonal sproutings due to their inability to maintain metabolic activity to the muscle fibers. The loss of muscle innervation results in decreased strength, endurance, and activity. Of those clients who have survived polio, 25% to 40% will experience the effects of post-polio syndrome.[1] Loss of lower extremity strength can result in clients overusing their upper extremities to compensate for their loss in function. Clients may begin to be unable to perform daily activities independently and may need to rely more on assistive devices and a wheelchair for mobility. A decrease in daily activities can result in weight gain, which is deleterious for maintaining independence in mobility.[2]

Comorbidities to Consider

• As the syndrome progresses, the client is likely to develop joint pain, myalgias, and fatigue, which may limit daily activities and independence with mobility tasks.

Client Examination

Keys to Examination of Clients

• Electromyograms and muscle biopsies are used to confirm loss of muscle innervation.
• Functional assessment of independence with transfers and gait may be appropriate for some clients.
• Employ a fatigue index to determine a baseline before having a client begin an exercise program.[3]

Recommended Baseline Testing of Fitness Levels

• Assess muscle strength with dynamometry using isometric and isokinetic resistance.
• Determine gait speed and independence using a 10-meter or 6-minute walk test.

Exercise Prescription

Type: Walking, treadmill walking, cycle ergometry, aquatic activities
Intensity: Low to moderate intensities, levels 12–15 on a Borg scale
Duration: Start at 10–15 minutes
Frequency: Three times per week

Getting Started

Prescribe an exercise program that matches the client's current level of function to prevent the client from experiencing excessive fatigue and muscle pain.[4] Endurance exercise using walking and treadmill walking is the most appropriate for promoting improvements in walking independence. Walking durations of up to 30 minutes, performed three times per week, have been used to improve endurance and to reduce fatigue levels.[5] Cycle ergometry and aquatics can be used to improve endurance and promote weight loss. Resistance exercise can be performed using a circuit of weight training, free weights, or resistance bands.[4,6] Resistance exercises can be prescribed with light to moderate resistance using one to three sets performed three times per week.[6] Regular participation in an exercise program is an important component for maintaining health, function, and quality of life in clients with post-polio syndrome.[1,2]

References

1. Post-Polio Health International. www.post-polio.org. Accessed Dec. 23, 2009.
2. Agre JC. The role of exercise in the patient with post-polio syndrome. Ann NY Acad Sci 753: 321-334, 1995.
3. Fatigue Severity Score. http://www.mult-sclerosis.org/fatigueseverityscale.html. Accessed November 24, 2009.
4. Abresch RT, Han JJ, Carter GT. Rehabilitation management of neuromuscular disease: The role of exercise training. J Clin Neuromuscul Dis 11(1):7-21, 2009.
5. Oncu J, Durmaz B, Karapolat H. Short-term effects of aerobic exercise on functional capacity, fatigue, and quality of life in patients with post-polio syndrome. Clin Rehabil 23(2):155-163, 2009.
6. Chan KM, Amirjani N, Sumrain M, et al. Randomized controlled trial of strength training in post-polio patients. Muscle Nerve 27(3):332-338, 2003.

RHABDOMYOLYSIS

Overview of Rhabdomyolysis

This condition is secondary to the breakdown of skeletal muscle fibers and seepage of the contents into the bloodstream. There are numerous causes, including traumatic crush, electrical injuries, ingestion of toxic substances, and exertional rhabdomyolysis, which occurs in endurance athletes and military personnel. A side effect of taking cholesterol-lowering statins can be the development of myopathies, which can progress to rhabdomyolysis.[1,2] The resulting complications include hyperkalemia, cardiac arrhythmias, and acute renal failure, which may lead to death. Early recognition of rhabdomyolysis will prevent the long-term complications from the loss of skeletal muscle and decreased renal and liver function.[3,4] Individuals who develop rhabdomyolysis will be counseled to avoid strenuous activities for a period of weeks to allow for return of kidney, liver, and cardiac function.[5] Individuals who have suffered heat overexertion may have long-term intolerance to heat/humidity conditions and decreased blood lactase thresholds.[4]

Comorbidities to Consider

- Clients may have suffered traumatic injuries or may develop renal and cardiac complications.

Client Examination

Keys to Examination of Clients

- Clients suspected of having this condition have urine samples tested for the presence of myoglobin or hemoglobin.
- Laboratory results for blood counts and levels of calcium, creatine kinase, sodium, and other contents are used in determining a client readiness to begin an exercise program.

Recommended Baseline Testing of Fitness Levels

- Endurance athletes can be assessed for their response to exercise using set workload parameters on a treadmill or cycle ergometer in a controlled environment for temperature and humidity. The athlete's heart rate and respiration can be monitored for response to increasing workloads, along with perceived exertion rates, to help establish a safe training program.[6] Athletes should be assessed for post-exercise muscle soreness and any changes to their urine output and appearance.
- Clients with traumatic injuries should be assessed for strength and mobility in involved muscle groups.
- Clients should be assessed for their functional levels to determine appropriate baseline tests.

Exercise Prescription

Type: Depends on the functional level of the client
Intensity: Low intensities with slow progressions
Duration: Varies
Frequency: Varies

Getting Started

Athletes who have developed rhabdomyolysis due to heat exertion illness should not participate in any strenuous activities for at least 1 week and must obtain clearance from their physician to return to training activities. Endurance athletes returning to their usual training activities should be encouraged to participate in a variety of activities to re-establish their training intensities with appropriate exertion levels. Exercise parameters will need to begin at levels that are low relative to the athlete's previous training levels. The athletes should avoid training in extreme heat conditions.[5] Environmental conditions must be carefully monitored and extreme conditions avoided until the athlete has demonstrated tolerance to full exertion and acclimitization.[7] Endurance athletes should take 4 to 6 weeks to return to their normal training levels and first pass a heat tolerance test.[5,8] Military personnel can return to usual activities with appropriate monitoring of their physiologic responses to exercise.[5,6]

Clients with traumatic injuries should begin with low-level strengthening activities, but they may have other musculoskeletal injuries that will restrict mobility and activities. Older athletes and untrained individuals should also start at low levels of exercise intensities and duration and monitor their response to the exercise program. Clients on statin drugs need ongoing assessment of their serum creatine kinase levels to determine when progression of strengthening exercises is appropriate.[1]

References

1. Venero CV, Thompson PD. Managing statin myopathy. Endocrinol Metab Clin North Am 38(1):121-136, 2009.
2. Tomlinson SS, Mangione KK. Potential adverse effects of statins on muscle. Phy Ther 85(5):459-465, 2005.
3. Sauret JM, Marinides G, Wang GK. Rhabdomyolysis. Am Fam Physician 65(5):907-912, 2002.
4. Hsu YD, Lee WH, Chang MK, et al. Blood lactate threshold and type II fibre predominance in patients with exertional heat stroke. J Neuro 62:182-187, 1997.
5. Armstrong LE, Casa DJ, Millard-Stafford D, et al. Exertional heat illness during training and competition. Med Sci Sports Exerc 39(3):556-572, 2007.
6. Armtrong LE, Lopez RM. Return to exercise training after heat exhaustion. J Sport Rehabil 16:182-189, 2007.
7. McDermott BP, Casa DJ, Yeargin SW, et al. Recovery and return to activity following exertional heat stroke: Considerations for the sports medicine staff. J Sport Rehabil 16:163-181, 2007.
8. Moran DS, Heled Y, Still Y, et al. Assessment of heat tolerance for post-exertional heat stroke individuals. Med Sci Monit 10:252-257, 2004.

RHEUMATOID ARTHRITIS

Overview of Rheumatoid Arthritis

This condition is a systemic, inflammatory disease that affects the articular and connective tissues. The disease process is characterized by periods of exacerbations and remissions. Clients develop progressive degeneration of articular structures, which lead to severe deformities and disabilities. The disease initially affects the joints of the hands, feet, and cervical spine. Progressions affect numerous tissues and organs, which may limit activities. During periods of exacerbations, clients experience severe limitations in mobility. Prolonged periods of rest result in joint pain and stiffness, which further reduce the client's activity level. The client may develop limited aerobic capacity, which affects endurance as the condition progresses.

Nonarticular Manifestations of Rheumatoid Arthritis

Anemia	Pericarditis
Neuropathies	Depression
Pulmonary effusions	Excessive fatigue

Comorbidities to Consider

- Clients may develop severe cervical instabilities and deformities of the hands, which may preclude participation in many exercise activities.

Client Examination

Keys to Examination of Clients

- Recent imaging studies of joint structures may help determine the progression of joint degeneration and connective tissue involvement.
- Assess the ankles and feet for signs of extensive degeneration, which may benefit from orthotics and assistive devices during exercise activities.

Recommended Baseline Testing of Fitness Levels

- Screen the client's posture, range of motion, and strength to determine general mobility.
- Measures of aerobic fitness can be assessed with walking or cycling tests.
- Condition-specific quality-of-life inventories, levels of fatigue, and depression are useful measures for determining the effects of an exercise program.[1]

Exercise Prescription

Type: Walking, cycling, recreational activities, weight training
Intensity: Low to moderate intensities
Duration: Start at 20 minutes
Frequency: Three to five times per week

Getting Started

Clients initially benefit most from a supervised exercise program that combines strengthening activities, aerobic training, and recreational activities.[1-5] Recreational activities of badminton, indoor soccer, basketball, volleyball, and step aerobics have been successfully used in group exercise sessions.[2] Clients' mobility and exercise tolerance will be greatly diminished during periods of exacerbations. Clients may experience temporary joint pain after participating in strength training. Joint pain that continues for longer than 1 hour would indicate that the exercise was excessive. Clients with extensive damage of large lower extremity joints should avoid activities that excessively load these joints.

Aerobic exercise of bicycle ergometer for 20 minutes at a perceived exertion level of 4 to 5 out of 10 is recommended along with 20 additional minutes of recreational activities. An intensive exercise program described by de Jong et al combines the effects of strength training and aerobic and recreational activities.[2] The strength training program used an exercise circuit of 8 to 10 exercises, using 8 to 15 repetitions for 20 minutes. Other exercise programs have used low-impact aerobic activities and walking to improve aerobic fitness and functional capacities.[1,6] Aquatic therapy, performed in water at least 35°C, using a combination of resistive and aerobic activities for 30 minutes is also recommended and may benefit clients who do not perceive the benefits of land-based exercises.[7] Clients can be progressed to independent programs with periodic consultations with a physical therapist to determine the most appropriate modes and parameters of exercise.

References

1. Neuberger GB, Aaronson LS, Gajewski B, et al. Predictors of exercise and effects of exercise on symptoms, function, aerobic fitness, and disease outcomes of rheumatoid arthritis. Arthritis Rheum 57(6):943-952, 2007.
2. de Jong Z, Munneke M, Zwinderman AH, et al. Is a long-term high-intensity exercise program effective and safe in patients with rheumatoid arthritis? Results of a randomized controlled trial. Arthritis Rheum 48(9):2415-2424, 2003.
3. Hsieh LF, Chen SC, Chuang CC, et al. Supervised aerobic exercise is more effective than home aerobic exercise in female Chinese patients with rheumatoid arthritis. J Rehabil Med 41(5):332-337, 2009.
4. van den Ende CH, Breedveld FC, le Cessie S, et al. Effect of intensive exercise on patients with active rheumatoid arthritis: A randomised clinical trial. Ann Rheum Dis 59(8):615-621, 2000.
5. Baillet A, Payraud E, Niderprim VA, et al. A dynamic exercise programme to improve patients' disability in rheumatoid arthritis: A prospective randomized controlled trial. Rheumatology (Oxford) 48(4):410-415, 2009.
6. Munnekem, de Jong Z, Zwinderman AH, et al. Effect of a high-intensity weight-bearing exercise program on radiologic damage progression of the large joints in subgroups of patients with rheumatoid arthritis. Arthritis Rheum 53(3):410-417, 2005.
7. Eversden L, Maggs F, Nightingale P, et al. A pragmatic randomised controlled trial of hydrotherapy and land exercises on overall well being and quality of life in rheumatoid arthritis. Musculoskeletal Disord 8:23, 2007.

SICKLE CELL DISEASE

Overview of Sickle Cell Disease

This disease is a group of inherited disorders that produces an abnormal type of hemoglobin that causes red blood cells to take on a sickle shape during deoxygenation. Sickling of red blood cells leads to lysis that results in anemia and vaso-occlusion. Sickled red blood cells form clots in organs, joints, and bones that produce painful episodes or crises. Sickle cell episodes can lead to damage to the spleen, with anemia leading to infections and systemic complications. Clients may have frequent crises that require ongoing medical management and complications. Infants are routinely screened for this disease. Clients are counseled to control their activities and stressors that may trigger a crises episode. Daily activities are difficult to complete if a client with sickle cell disease has chronic anemia.[1,2]

Comorbidities to Consider

- Determine if the client has anemia or other systemic complications of this disease process.

Client Examination

Keys to Examination of Clients

- Assess the results of blood tests for hematocrit and hemoglobin levels and reticulocyte and white blood cell counts as well as tests for liver and renal function.
- Perform a thorough medical history to understand clients' history of sickling crises and the complications from the disease process.
- Determine if clients have any persistent joint or mobility problems.

Recommended Baseline Testing of Fitness Levels

- A 1-mile or 6-minute walk test can be an appropriate method for assessing clients' aerobic fitness and tolerance to endurance activities.[2]

Exercise Prescription

Type: Aerobic and recreational activities
Intensity: Brief episodes of high-intensity activities
Duration: Varies
Frequency: Three to seven times per week

Getting Started

Aerobic activities and recreational activities are most appropriate for these clients and should begin at low intensities. Clients should consider their exercise activity to be enjoyable and not an excessive stressor to their lifestyle. Young children may choose to participate in activities that require brief episodes of sprinting, such as soccer or baseball, and will need to rest when they feel fatigued.[1,3] Young people should be encouraged to participate in school and recreational activities to allow for normal development and normal social interactions.[3,4] They will need to be able to rest when fatigued and have regular access to hydration. They will need more time for acclimation to excessive heat, cold, and higher-altitude conditions. They should avoid long periods of underwater swimming or scuba diving.[1,4]

References

1. Nemours Foundation: Teens Health from Nemours. Sickle Cell Anemia. http://kidshealth.org/parent/medical/heart/sickle_cell_anemia.html#. Accessed August 30, 2009.
2. Liem RI, Nevin MA, Prestridge A, et al. Functional capacity in children and young adults with sickle cell disease undergoing evaluation for cardiopulmonary disease. Am J Hematol 84(10):645-649, 2009.
3. Al-Rimawi H, Jallad S. Sport participation in adolescents with sickle cell disease. Pediatr Endocrinol Rev 6(Suppl 1):214-216, 2008.
4. Sickle Cell Society: Information for Health Professionals. http://www.sicklecellsociety.org/pdf/SC4.pdf. Accessed August 30, 2009.

SICKLE CELL TRAIT

Overview of Sickle Cell Trait

This is an inherited condition of abnormal hemoglobin production. This condition rarely results in a sickling crisis and is managed differently from sickle cell disease. An exertional sickling crisis usually occurs when athletes or military personnel with this condition overexert themselves, resulting in sickling of red blood cells, which causes clotting and ischemic rhabdomyolysis.[1] Most individuals with sickle cell trait do not have painful crises and can participate in regular recreational and competitive activities, but abnormalities of red blood cell parameters may influence their aerobic exercise tolerance.[2,3] Dehydration, viral illness, abrupt changes in altitude, and exercising in heat conditions are risk factors for developing exertional sickling.[1,4]

Comorbidities to Consider

- Clients with this condition may have temporary states of anemia and develop complications if they develop rhabdomyolysis.

Client Examination

Keys to Examination of Clients

- If sickling crises occurs, monitor hemoglobin levels and renal function before allowing a return to strenuous training and competitive activities.[4]
- Screen athletes for this condition so that if a crisis occurs, it can be identified and treated as a medical emergency.

Recommended Baseline Testing of Fitness Levels

- Competitive athletes with this condition may choose to be tested for the rate of red blood cell sickling during strenuous exercise to better understand their risk for developing an exertional sickling crises.[1]

Exercise Prescription

Type: Aerobic and recreational activities
Intensity: No limitations
Duration: No limitations
Frequency: No limitations

Getting Started

Clients can choose to participate in any type of recreational or competitive pursuits, but they should have proper conditioning to participate in activities and should be counseled on how to recognize symptoms of a sickling crisis.[1] Counsel them to avoid all-out exertion of any activity for longer than 3 minutes and to use rest periods with full recovery when performing interval training.[1] Clients should properly hydrate during exercise and adjust training programs for hot and humid conditions. They should be counseled to increase their training programs slowly to acclimatize to temperature, humidity, and altitude.[1]

References

1. Eichner ER. Sickle Cell Trait. J Sports Rehabil 16(3);197-203, 2007.
2. Connes P, Reid H, Hardy-Dessources MD, et al. Physiological responses of sickle cell trait carriers during exercise. Sports Med 38(11):931-946, 2008.
3. Connes P, Hue O, Tripette J, et al. Blood rheology abnormalities and vascular cell adhesion mechanisms in sickle cell trait carriers during exercise. Clin Hemorheol Microcirc 39:179-184, 2008.
4. Markaryus JN, Catanzaro JN, Katona KC. Exertional rhabdomyolysis and renal failure in patients with sickle cell trait: Is it time to change our approach? Hematology 12(4):349-352, 2007.

SLEEP APNEA SYNDROME

Overview of Sleep Apnea Syndrome

This disorder causes interrupted sleep patterns and respiratory gas exchange. The syndrome results in significant daytime sleepiness due to upper airway obstruction and sleep disturbances. The three types of sleep apnea are obstructive, central, and mixed. Obstructive apnea results from collapse of the pharyngeal tissues, and central apnea results from decreased cerebral respiratory control. Sleep apnea syndrome is related to obesity, large neck circumference, eating disorders, depression, and sedentary activity levels. Clients are commonly treated with continuous positive airway pressure during sleep. Clients do not attain deep restorative sleep, which results in daytime fatigue, headaches, and cognitive impairments. The lack of regular exercise has been associated with increased levels of sleep apnea.[1]

Comorbidities to Consider

• Clients may also have a history of hypertension, thyroid conditions, and seizure disorders.

Client Examination

Keys to Examination of Clients

• Clients are diagnosed through overnight polysomnography to monitor sleep patterns and blood oxygen saturation.
• The apnea-hypopnea or respiratory disturbance index (RDI) is determined based on the number of cessations of breathing occurring per hour of sleep.[2]
• Clients' RDI can help classify their level of sleep apnea, and daily levels of sleepiness can be assessed with the Epworth Sleepiness Scale.[3,4]

Respiratory Disturbance Index

Mild: 5–15 sleep disturbances per hour
Moderate: 15–30 sleep disturbances per hour
Severe: More than 30 disturbances per hour

Recommended Baseline Testing of Fitness Levels

• Use a walking test to assess cardiorespiratory function and aerobic fitness
• Clients may have hypertension and other heart disease–related conditions that will require frequent monitoring during exercise programs.

Exercise Prescription

Type: Walking, treadmill walking, cycling
Intensity: Low to moderate intensities
Duration: 20–30 minutes
Frequency: Three to five times per week

Getting Started

Exercise programs should be used as an adjunct treatment strategy for patients with mild to moderate obstructive sleep apnea, as limited evidence exists for the efficacy of exercise programs improving sleep apnea.[5,6] Aerobic activities of walking, treadmill walking, or cycling with the goal of improving RDI and daytime sleepiness and reducing body adipose tissues and health risk factors should be the main mode of exercise. Clients should also be encouraged to make moderate reductions in their daily caloric intake.

Aerobic exercise prescription based on a patient's age and baseline fitness should be used to start the exercise program. Clients should be encouraged to exercise daily at low to moderate intensity levels with a goal of 150 to 250 minutes of total physical activity per week, or 1500 to 1800 kcal of physical activities along with appropriate caloric intake limits, to bring about weight loss.[7,8] Clients may not tolerate activities in supine positions due to breathing difficulties even when awake. Because clients have found self-initiated exercises difficult to maintain, their intention to exercise should be assessed, and counseling may be needed to progress the client to a preparation and action stage of behavior change.[9] Clients' exercise program frequency and duration should be progressed to attain weight loss goals. Clients should be counseled to maintain a regular exercise program to maintain weight loss and reduce health risk factors associated with sleep apnea.

References

1. Peppard PE, Young T. Exercise and sleep-disordered breathing: An association independent of body habitus. Sleep 27(3):480-484, 2004.
2. Redline S, Budhiraja R, Kapur VJ. The scoring of respiratory events in sleep: Reliability and validity. Clin Sleep Med 3(2):169-200, 2007.
3. Epworth Sleepiness Scale. http://www.stanford.edu/~dement/epworth.html. Accessed November 25, 2009.
4. Johns MW. Sleepiness in different situations measured by the Epworth Sleepiness Scale. Sleep 17:703-710, 1994.
5. Giebelhaus V, Strohl KP, Lormes W, et al. Physical exercise as an adjunct therapy in sleep apnea: An open trial. Sleep Breathing 4(4):173-176, 2000.
6. Norman JF, Von Essen SG, Fuchs RH. Exercise training effect on obstructive sleep apnea syndrome. Sleep Res Online. 3(3):121-129, 2000.
7. Stiegler P, Cunliffe A. The role of diet and exercise for the maintenance of fat-free mass and resting metabolic rate during weight loss. Sports Med 36(3):239-262, 2006.
8. Donnelly JE, Blair SN, Jakicic JM, et al. American College of Sports Medicine position stand: Appropriate physical activity intervention strategies for weight loss and prevention of weight regain for adults. Med Sci Sports Exerc 41(2):459-471, 2009.
9. Smith SS, Doyle G, Pascoe T, et al. Intention to exercise in patients with obstructive sleep apnea. J Clin Sleep Med 3(7):686-694, 2007.

SLEEP DISORDERS, AGE-RELATED

Overview of Age-Related Sleep Disorders

Sleep disorders are commonly associated with the effects of aging. Aging affects the levels of melatonin and growth hormones, which help regulate arousal and sleep cycles. Medications taken for chronic conditions can also affect sleep cycles. Individuals who have difficulty falling asleep or staying asleep for adequate periods may use excessive chemical substances to help produce sleep and then use other substances to enhance their arousal and attention during the day.[1] Individuals who work rotating shift hours or travel across time zones may find adapting to changes in their sleep cycle more difficult as they age. Sleep disorders affect mood, attention levels, and concentration during waking hours. Clients with sleep disorders may not feel they have enough energy or stamina to participate in regular exercise programs.[2]

Comorbidities to Consider

- Client may have mood disorders and cardiovascular diseases that are also associated with aging.

Client Examination

Keys to Examination of Clients

- A sleep polysomnographic test is used to assess the stages of sleep that these clients attain and the number of awakenings during the night.
- Perform baseline assessments of posture, balance, and flexibility before developing an exercise program for a client.
- Employ a questionnaire, such as the Epworth Sleepiness Scale, to assess sleep quality and daytime sleepiness.[3]

Recommended Baseline Testing of Fitness Levels

- Aerobic capacity can be assessed with submaximal tests using walking and cycle ergometry.
- Screen for cardiopulmonary risk factors and risks for falling before starting a new exercise program.

Exercise Prescription

Type: Walking, bicycling, aquatherapy, and tai chi[4-6]
Intensity: Moderate intensities of 60%–85% of peak heart rate
Duration: Start at 30 minutes
Frequency: 5 days per week

Getting Started

Exercises to improve sleep quality are generally recommended to be done in the morning and outdoors, as evening exercise may interfere with the circadian rhythms and body temperatures to promote sleep.[2] Aerobic exercise increasing to 45 minutes for 5 days per week have been shown to have the best treatment response for improving sleep quality.[5,7] The combination of aerobic exercise with stretching, resistive exercise and coordination activities for improving balance are also recommended for these individuals. Clients should be encouraged to increase the duration and frequency of their exercise programs gradually to maintain 5 days per week for 45 minutes.[5]

References

1. Misra S, Malow BA. Evaluation of sleep disturbances in older adults. Clin Geriatr Med 24(1):15-26, 2008.
2. Youngstedt SD. Effects of exercise on sleep. Clin Sports Med 24:355-365, 2005.
3. Johns MW. Sleepiness in different situations measured by the Epworth Sleepiness Scale. Sleep 17:703-710, 1994.
4. Irwin MR, Olmstead R, Motivala SJ. Improving sleep quality in older adults with moderate sleep complaints: A randomized controlled trial of tai chi. Sleep 31(7):1001-1008, 2008.
5. King AC, Pruitt LA, Woo S, et al. Effects of moderate-intensity exercise on polysomnographic and subjective sleep quality in older adults with mild to moderate sleep complaints. J Gerontol A Biol Sci Med Sci 63A:997-1004, 2008.
6. Li F, Fisher KJ, Harmer P et al. Tai chi and self-rated quality of sleep and daytime sleepiness in older adults: A randomized controlled trial. J Am Geriatr Soc 52(6):892-900, 2004.
7. Tworoger SS, Yasui Y, Vitiello MV, et al. Effects of a year-long moderate-intensity exercise and a stretching intervention on sleep quality in postmenopausal women. Sleep 26(7):830-836, 2003.

TUBERCULOSIS

Overview of Tuberculosis

Tuberculosis is an infectious disease that affects the lungs and can spread to the lymph nodes and other organs. It is caused by the mycobacterium tuberculosis, which creates necrotic granulomas in the parenchyma of the lungs. The tissues of the lungs control these organisms by forming a tubercle around the infection. Individuals with this condition usually are asymptomatic until they become debilitated due to another illness that results in a depressed immune system. The infection then spreads through the lobes of the lungs and becomes systemic through the lymph nodes. Clients exhibit a chronic productive cough, crackles (formerly called rales), and bronchial breath sounds, with fever, weight loss, and malaise. They have signs of excessive inflammation and exudates from their lungs that make breathing difficult. The infection can spread to numerous other tissues (including bone), resulting in their destruction. Clients with the spread of infection into connective tissues experience limited mobility and pain. Clients with an active tuberculosis episode have limited endurance due to their inflammatory lung condition.

Comorbidities to Consider

- Clients whose status is post-tuberculosis have lung damage that creates a restrictive lung disease and possibly a chronic obstructive pulmonary disease.[1]

Client Examination

Keys to Examination of Clients

- The tuberculin skin test and QuantiFERON-TB blood tests are used to diagnose this condition, and a chest radiograph is taken for the location and size of the tubercle.
- Clients in a post-tuberculosis state have restricted lung capacities and may have altered trunk postures, muscle weakness, and breathing patterns that affect their tolerance to endurance activities.[2]
- Assessment of rib cage and extremity mobility help determine the types of interventions that are most appropriate.

Recommended Baseline Testing of Fitness Levels

- A 6-minute walk test is recommended before starting a pulmonary rehabilitation program.
- Clients whose status is post-tuberculosis should be assessed for dyspnea and lung function testing.

Exercise Prescription

Type: Walking, stationary cycling, and weight training
Intensity: Low intensities
Duration: 20–30 minutes
Frequency: 5–6 days per week

Getting Started

Exercises can include endurance activities, strength training for proximal upper and lower extremity muscles, and diaphragmatic breathing exercises. Supervised endurance activities of walking or treadmill walking and stationary bicycling are appropriate for beginning the exercise program. Exercise intensity is best assessed by the client's perceived exertion levels and by ratings of dyspnea. For strength training, use a circuit of free weights and pulley exercises at low intensities, with 12 to 20 repetitions for up to 30 minutes. Diaphragmatic breathing training can be performed in supine and sitting positions with an emphasis on rib cage expansion and controlled expirations with pursed lip breathing.[2] Clients can be seen one to two times per week for supervised exercise sessions, with home exercise activities two to four times per week. Clients should be encouraged to develop and maintain a home program of endurance and strengthening activities to maintain their quality of life and a healthy immune response.[3]

References

1. Phillips MS, Kinnear WJ, Shaw D, et al. Exercise responses in patients treated for pulmonary tuberculosis by thoracoplasty. Thorax 44:268-274, 1989.
2. Ando M, Mori A, Esaki H, et al. The effect of pulmonary rehabilitation in patients with post-tuberculosis lung disorder. Chest 123:1988-1995, 2003.
3. Okutsu M, Yoshida Y, Zhang X, et al. Exercise training enhances in vivo tuberculosis purified protein derivative response in the elderly. J Appl Physiol 104(6):1690-1696, 2008.

Index